Every
You

CW00956434

REVOLUTIONARY ASTHMA TREATMENT

Every Breath You Take

DR PAUL J. AMEISEN

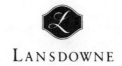

LANSDOWNE

*To those who over-breathe — may they
normalise their breathing so that they each
breathe for one person*

Published by Lansdowne Australia Pty Ltd
PO Box 48 Millers Point, Sydney NSW 2000, Australia

Publisher: Cheryl Hingley
Creative Director: Sally Stokes

First published by Lansdowne Publishing 1997

Designed by Susanne Geppert
Diagrams by Tina Watson
Printed by McPherson's Printing Group, Victoria, Australia

National Library of Australia Cataloguing-in-Publication Data

Ameisen Paul J.
Every breath you take

Includes index.
ISBN 1 86302 567 7.

1. Asthma - Treatment - Popular works. 2. Breathing
exercises - Therapeutic use. I. Title.

Contents

Introduction 6

Effective Treatment for Asthma 14
The Buteyko Method

Practising the Method 28
Step by Step — How People Learn to
Breathe Correctly

A New Lease of Life 44
Former Asthma Sufferers Tell Their Stories

How Does the Buteyko Method Work? 86
The Physiology of Breathing

Treatment of Asthma with Drugs 106
Current Approaches

Asthma and Naturopathy 126
Other Treatments for Asthma

The Buteyko Method in Russia 144

The Buteyko Method in Other Countries 154

Appendices 180
A Letter from Professor Buteyko

*Some Common Questions about the Method,
and the Answers*

Acknowledgments 190
Index 194

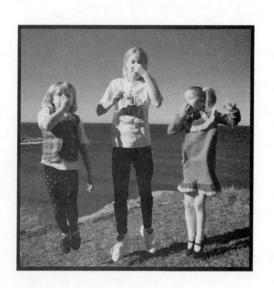

Introduction

I have been a medical practitioner for twenty-one years, with both city and country practices, and in that time I have treated thousands of asthma patients. Like every conscientious medical doctor I have kept up-to-date with the latest research, and with advances in techniques and medication, in order to help my patients to the best of my ability. This has been especially important to me, as I take a keen interest in respiratory diseases. In addition, my work has been in Australia, where a major respiratory disease has a strong hold: Australia and New Zealand have more asthma sufferers per capita than any other country in the world. More than one million people have asthma in Australia (some estimate nearly two million) — that is, 25% of children, 15% of teenagers and 10% of adults have asthma.

Asthma is on the increase in the industrialised countries of the world. In the USA, 16 million people suffer

OPPOSITE PAGE: *The Buteyko technique for the treatment of asthma is so natural it can even be fun.*

from it, and three million in the United Kingdom. Boys have asthma more commonly than girls in childhood and about one child in four has asthma at some stage of development. About half of the children with mild asthma will improve and 'grow out of' the condition through their teenage years. The others have to continue with a disease that can interfere with their pleasure in life, their education, their sporting interests, their well-being and even their relationships with family and friends. Adult or 'late onset' asthma also occurs, more frequently in women than in men. These unlucky people not only suffer acute discomfort, disruption of every aspect of their lives and often sheer misery from their condition, but they may also be facing a threat to their life. Not only asthma itself, but deaths from asthma attacks are on the increase. In Australia in 1996, for instance, it is a frightening fact that asthma attacks caused more than 800 deaths.

Medicine in the twentieth century has not coped well with asthma. The number and availability of drugs to treat the disease have been sharply increasing since the beginning of the century — but so has the incidence of asthma. The Asthma Foundation of Australia reported that the incidence of asthma in children in Australia actually doubled between 1982 and 1992. As a doctor I could not help wishing that there was another way of helping a child control his or her asthma, instead of having to fall back on an increase in the drugs I prescribed.

Then, more than six years ago, I first became aware of the work and methods of a certain Professor Konstantin

Pavlovich Buteyko, a diagnostic physician whose techniques were considered a breakthrough in Russia, after a lifetime of research and treatment of asthma patients. It was two of my patients who told me about it — a mother and daughter who had attended a clinic in Sydney and had both derived extraordinary benefit from the simple breathing technique that they were taught by the Buteyko practitioner.

I became interested, and I observed the technique over a long period. Doctors are always cautious about any new research or treatments they observe, and I was no exception. But there is nothing more convincing to a scientific mind than genuine, sustained and verifiable results and I eventually became convinced, from the objective evidence, that I was looking at a dramatically effective treatment for asthma. I began referring patients to the clinic and became supervising medical officer, which enabled me to monitor and help my patients and others even more effectively. Consequently I have also been able to make a study of the 8,000 patients treated so far in Australia, and when invited I have spoken on radio and television about the far-reaching beneficial effects of this natural, benign method. My book is the result of six years of research into the method and the results it has achieved for asthma sufferers.

The results are astonishing and suggest a direct link between our breathing patterns and our level of health. The Buteyko theory is that the basic cause of asthma is habitual, hidden over-breathing (literally taking in too much air when we breathe). The treatment is based on bringing the breathing to normal levels and thus eradicating over-breathing (hyperventilation), and reversing the need for the body's defence mechanisms. These defence mechanisms, according to the theory, include: spasm of the airways; mucus production (chest, nose, throat and ears); inflammation (swelling) of the bronchial walls. These defence mechanisms are fully explained in the chapter 'How Does the Buteyko Method Work?'.

The message of the Buteyko method is that when asthma sufferers learn to alter the volume of air they habitually inhale, their asthma attacks can be significantly reduced and the use of asthma drugs and apparatus can be reduced or entirely eliminated.

It is possible that the economies of the industrialised countries worldwide could save billions of dollars spent annually on asthma drug subsidies and hospitalisation, if their health administrators took notice of the advances in asthma treatment pioneered by Professor Buteyko. It is on record as having benefited 100,000 patients in Russia, and is officially recognised by the Russian government. Professor Buteyko's experimentation and clinical trials on documented patients in Russia indicate that the great majority of asthma sufferers over four years old can be significantly relieved by the method, and any individual on asthma drug treatment can reduce that drug intake by 90% or more in a majority of cases.

Outside Russia, the first Buteyko clinical trials on asthma sufferers were completed in 1995 in Australia by

Associate Professor Charles Mitchell of the Queensland University Medical School, Dr Simon Bowler of the Mater Hospital and Ms Tess Graham of the Buteyko Group.

The results of the first half of the trial, which were presented to a conference of the Thoracic Society in Hobart on March 30, 1995, supported the findings of Professor Buteyko, and a press release at the time made the general findings public. The Buteyko method is available in all capital cities in Australia and has spread to workshops in country areas. The statistics of more than 8,000 cases so far (1997) in Australia show that the success rate continues to be very high. Asthma sufferers attending the clinics have found that after learning and practising the method they can reduce the use of their relievers and preventers to varying significant degrees. As I write this Introduction, the positive results of the clinical analysis of the method carried out in Queensland are due for publication.

It is impossible to overestimate the importance of the Buteyko method for asthma sufferers and their families. I believe it is the great medical breakthrough of the twentieth century, and I am proud to be able to offer the first ever book on this subject outside Russia. This book is the result of my own investigation of the theory and practice of the method, and relies on my close experience of the clinics and the patients who have benefited from them, over the last six years. I have the sanction of Professor Buteyko and of the Buteyko clinics to reveal the method, its scientific bases and its results.

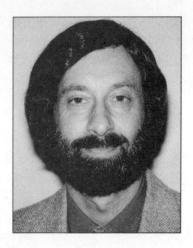

Dr Paul Ameisen has been a Medical Practitioner for twenty-one years. His first appointment was as Resident at St Vincents Hospital, Sydney, and he has since practised at Liverpool Hospital, Framingham Union Hospital in Boston, USA; Baragwanath Hospital, South Africa; Mudgee District Hospital, NSW. He has a Diploma of Naturopathy, a Diploma Medicina Alternativa, and is a Fellow of the Australian College of Nutritional and Environmental Medicine.

This book is not a self-teach manual, since a practitioner and a doctor are necessary to monitor each person's progress and give advice as to whether their medication can be safely reduced or stopped. One chapter of this book is devoted to a step-by-step description of the breathing technique itself: the chapter is not an instruction manual, as the method must be taught by a trained teacher.

Thus, through this book, asthma sufferers and the millions of others who may suffer the hidden effects of over-breathing have an opportunity to assess all the aspects of the method and all the relevant medical background, and to decide whether they would like to eventually learn the technique for their own benefit, or share the discovery with others.

I have great pleasure and confidence in recommending this technique to all asthma sufferers and all practitioners — medical, paramedical, orthodox and complementary.

I am delighted to offer this book to the public, because it is the first time all the facts about the method have been available to everyone, as I believe they should be.

Paul J. Ameisen
MBBS, ND, Dip Ac,
FACNEM

January 1997

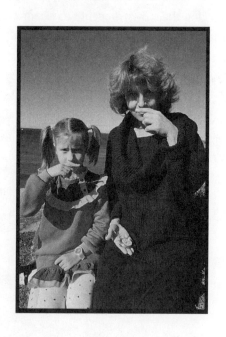

Effective Treatment for Asthma

The Buteyko Method

This chapter takes a look into the lungs to give a simple explanation of Professor Buteyko's theory concerning the underlying cause of asthma, what is believed to trigger it, and how it can be treated most effectively.

The fourth chapter, 'How Does the Buteyko Method Work?', gives the full medical theory behind the method, with diagrams and graphs, and the scientifically minded may well wish to turn there first.

Here I offer a broad view, which will help asthma sufferers to understand the research and the theory, both of which concern the way we breathe. Basically, the idea of the Buteyko exercises is to restore healthy breathing, because this is the key to controlling asthma.

I also want to give hope and inspiration to the families of asthma sufferers, especially the parents of asthmatic children, who have been searching for a natural answer to the problems and anxiety they face.

OPPOSITE PAGE: *The only equipment required to practise the Buteyko method is a stopwatch.*

We Need Carbon Dioxide

You may have thought that in a discussion about the lungs we would talk about oxygen first and foremost. But the first thing I want to bring up here is how important carbon dioxide is in the body. In fact we know that each human cell needs *a specific concentration of carbon dioxide — about 7%* — to sustain normal life.

When human life first began on the planet, the composition of the atmosphere was different from what it is today — there was more than 20% of carbon dioxide in the air that living beings breathed. But by now the percentage has fallen greatly — our air contains only 0.03% of carbon dioxide. Our bodies have had to gradually compensate for this, and they have done so by creating an *internal air environment* in the small air sacs inside the lungs. With the action of normal, healthy breathing, these air sacs contain around 6.5% of carbon dioxide.

So, as we breathe in and out normally, that 6.5% of carbon dioxide exists inside the lungs, in balance with the oxygen that we also need to stay alive.

An important factor that seriously affects that level of necessary carbon dioxide in the lungs is *over-breathing*, also known as *hyperventilation*. If we breathe in too great a volume of air for our body's needs, we breathe off carbon dioxide too rapidly, and the lungs are unable to maintain the right level in the air sacs. When carbon dioxide is low due to over-breathing, this causes a chemical reaction which makes it hard for oxygen to be released from the blood stream into the tissues of the body. The *tissues of the body then become starved of oxygen*.

Tissues starved of oxygen cannot be healthy: they become irritable, and smooth muscles react by going into *spasm*. Smooth muscle is found around our air tubes and around blood vessels, arteries and veins, and forms part of the wall of the intestines.

Oxygen starvation of vital organs (such as the brain) excites the breathing centre in the brain, thereby creating a state of *breathing stimulation*. This increases the breathing even further, creating a 'shortness of breath' sensation in the already deep-breathing person, which further deepens the breath and creates a vicious circle, because we breathe off even more carbon dioxide.

What Are The Results of Over-breathing?

This century, a Russian respiratory physician, Professor Buteyko, came up with the theory that a majority of the human population actually over-breathes — some more severely than others. Because people are unaware of this factor, he called it *hidden hyperventilation* — long-term over-breathing not clearly visible to the individual.

He noticed that the result of obvious over-breathing has the equivalent effect of an acute and serious anxiety

BREATHING LEVELS

Normal breathing	3 to 5 litres per minute	Healthy level of 6.5% carbon dioxide in air sacs
Hidden over-breathing	5 to 10 litres per minute	Results in very gradual sickness not easily noticed, and illness develops over many years
Over-breathing	10 to 20 litres per minute	This is known as an 'attack', where the adult asthma sufferer, or a person with a related condition, hyperventilates rapidly
Severe over-breathing	20 to 30 litres per minute	At this maximum level, the person suffers a sudden anxiety attack

attack — shaking hands, anxiety, chest pain, air hunger, finger tingles and spasm (tetany), cramps, racing pulse. He went on to believe that the effect of less serious over-breathing, which is not noticed immediately, has equally dire consequences for a person's health, over time.

The amount of air we breathe is measured in litres. The table shows the effects of normal breathing and over-breathing.

In general the person's system becomes ill through over-breathing, and is then more prone to viral illness and allergies. The shift in the rate of body activity disturbs the normal flow of chemical reactions in the body and further illness results.

If over-breathing disturbs our basic total metabolism, as the Professor believes, we can start to understand how it might cause a diverse set of symptoms: bronchospasm (spasming of the air tubes), heart blood vessel spasm, and increased blood pressure. These symptoms are recognised and help us define certain diseases: *asthma*, angina, hypertension. Professor Buteyko concluded that these in turn, if breathing is not corrected, lead to further *deterioration of asthma*, sclerosis (hardening) of blood vessels and lungs, myocardial infarction (heart attack) and strokes. The Buteyko theory states that these diseases are the body's defence mechanism against the excessive loss of carbon dioxide through over-breathing.

The chapter 'How Does the Buteyko Method Work?' goes into the medical facts about the body's activity in general, and the other diseases. Here we will concentrate on breathing and asthma. For this, it is important to remember that the human organism tries at all times to keep carbon dioxide at the normal, beneficial level in the lungs. When we over-breathe, therefore, Buteyko explains that the body adopts a defence mechanism to retain carbon dioxide. These are signs of this at work:

1. Spasm of the airways and air sacs: they close up to make openings narrower, in an effort to keep the carbon dioxide in the lungs.

2. Mucus and phlegm develop: this is another way for the body to narrow the airways in an attempt to trap the carbon dioxide.

3. Swelling of the mucus lining and the bronchial tubes: a further way for the body to narrow the airways.

Asthma sufferers will instantly recognise the above symptoms. There is another that is not obvious to those who over-breathe:

4. Increased production of cholesterol in the liver, which causes a thickening of the cell walls of the blood vessels, which in turn prevents loss of carbon dioxide from the blood vessels back to the small air sacs in the lungs.

Professor Buteyko concluded that to avoid making the body ill through over-breathing, and also to avoid the uncomfortable and unpleasant effects of the defence mechanism at work, the solution was to educate the over-breathers so that they could learn to breathe in a shallower way — so that the lungs could return to normality, that is, keep the carbon dioxide level at around 6.5%.

To achieve this re-education, it was important for people to see what factors were making them over-breathe in the first place.

Triggers That Are Considered to Cause Over-breathing

1. The belief that deep breathing is helpful and improves health. This is received wisdom in the Western world, though not in Eastern cultures, where shallow breathing is practised for bodily and mental health. We breathe in more air when we exercise, it is true — but it does not follow that regular deep breathing is beneficial. In fact, try to make the barbecue fire catch by breathing in deeply and blowing out hard, and you will rapidly become faint. Observe top athletes and swimmers — these super fit people have the slowest pulse and shallowest breathing in the population. A fit, healthy body breathes slowly and more shallowly. Swimming is the best sport for asthma sufferers, because swimmers hold their breath while exercising — they practise the Buteyko method without realising it.

2. Stress: from both positive and negative emotions. Both excitement and depression cause stress, and research shows that people under stress over-breathe.

3. Over-eating. When we eat too much the system has to work harder to process the food, and this can cause over-breathing. To avoid this one should not over-eat. It is also a fact that animal protein makes the body work harder. Many asthma sufferers will have noticed that red meat and cheese, for example (animal protein) sharply increase hyperventilation. To avoid over-breathing caused by the food we eat, it is better to eat more plant products than animal products. You should also eat raw food more than cooked food (raw food causes less over-breathing).

4. Lack of regular exercise. Physical activity on the other hand encourages the release of carbon dioxide from the body cells, increasing its level in the lungs. In vigorous exercise (except for swimming) of course we breathe deeply, and this results in a short-term drop in carbon dioxide; but the long-term result of fitness is a higher level of carbon dioxide in the lungs and better nourishment of all the cells in the body.

5. Prolonged, excessive sleep. Professor Buteyko's research demonstrates that lying down for a long time, especially on the back, while asleep or while bed-ridden, causes severe over-breathing. Techniques to avoid over-breathing in horizontal positions are described in the next chapter. Patients should sleep only 6–7 hours if possible, on the left side, and breathe through the nose, with the mouth firmly shut.

6. Hot and stuffy environments. We over-breathe when our body detects that the air we are breathing does not contain what we need. On the other hand, mild or cold temperatures all assist shallow breathing — a conclusion reached over 40 years of research and measurement. We soon realise this when we sit in a sauna. Sweating may detoxify the body, but it also creates extra work, causing hyperventilation. When we move from a cooler climate to a hot one, a similar reaction can occur.

7. Bronchodilators. These are standard medication for asthmatics. Bronchodilators give quick relief at first, but Buteyko argues that they in fact cause further over-breathing — because they are designed to open the air passages and maximally keep them open for four to twelve hours, allowing the sufferer to continue what he or she thinks of as 'normal' breathing. Based on Professor Buteyko's research, a person who suffers from asthma is an over-breather — so after two to twelve hours the low carbon dioxide means that the airways will go into spasm again, and the bronchodilator will be needed once more — a vicious circle.

8. Excessive sexual activity. The hyperventilation in sexual activity is obvious — and normal. It is only when this activity becomes excessive because of a sex addiction that hyperventilation becomes a problem, because it lowers the level of carbon dioxide in the lungs.

9. Smoking and pollution. When we walk into a smoke-filled room we may cough — this is because we are entering a situation that is allergic and toxic. We also get the signal 'not enough air', so we over-breathe.

Some people — asthmatics included — react more sensitively to such situations than others, and have the same reaction to pollution, which causes over-breathing.

10. Alcohol and recreational drugs. These put a stress on the body due to their toxicity and overstimulation, and Professor Buteyko's studies give evidence that they lead to over-breathing.

The Aim of the Buteyko Method

The aim is to use a series of regulated breathing exercises to teach the person who over-breathes to breathe a normal volume of air for the rest of his or her life. An adult who suffers from asthma usually breathes 5 to 10 litres of air a minute when he or she is 'well'. During an attack, the rate increases to 10 to 20 litres per minute. The simple, and achievable, aim of the method is to get the volume of air down to normal — 3 to 4 litres per minute. It can be done — thousands of relieved patients have proved it — and the technique is so simple a child can follow the method, and even have fun while learning.

As you will see from the chapter entitled 'A New Lease of Life', the joy of former asthma sufferers, once they have mastered the technique and returned their breathing and their lives to normal, is overwhelming.

Symptoms that patients may suffer from prior to commencing the Buteyko course

Over-breathing leads to different ailments in different people, depending on their susceptibility. People who suffer from severe asthma, to the extent that they are regularly hospitalised and have to cope with a much deteriorated state of health, may suffer from a variety of symptoms. Below is a list of those that have been noted by Buteyko practitioners, in a wide variety of individuals.

* Headache
* Dizziness
* Insomnia
* Loss of memory
* Mental fatigue
* Irritability
* Fear of sultry air
* Lack of concentration
* Loss of smell

* Diarrhoea
* Shortness of breath
* Breathing through mouth
* Frequent deep breaths
* Tightness around chest
* Short temper
* Rhinitis
* Trembling and tic

- Fear without reason
- Apathy
- Coughing
- Loss of feeling in the limbs
- Impotence
- Dryness in the mouth
- Deterioration of vision
- Far-sightedness
- Allergies
- Chest pain (not around heart)
- Sudden chill of limbs and other parts
- Asthma attacks
- Dysmenorrhoea (painful periods)
- Menorrhagia (heavy periods)
- Muscle pains
- Deterioration of hearing
- Prone to colds or flu
- Flashes before the eyes
- Shuddering in sleep
- Sterility
- Frigidity
- Pains in heart region
- Unusual weight gain
- Unusual weight loss
- Bleeding veins
- Varicose veins
- Sudden physical exhaustion
- Pains in the bones
- Anaemia
- Itching
- Dry skin

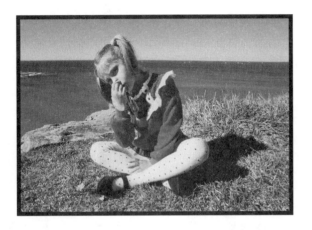

Practising the Method

Step by Step — How People Learn to Breathe Correctly

This chapter reveals all the steps of the Buteyko method, which is designed to ensure that anyone who practises it can learn to breathe normally. At this point it is necessary to issue a warning to the reader, more especially to asthma patients who are already undergoing treatment for asthma, whether with drugs or not.

This chapter is not intended as an instruction manual to teach the technique. The method must be taught by a specially trained teacher, as there are many variations and nuances. When a person masters the technique, the degree to which he or she reduces (or eventually even drops) the medication must be directed and monitored by the teacher and the patient's doctor.

All patients who attend Buteyko clinics must bring their medication to all classes. You will see by reading the case histories in the next chapter how the method improves patients' health and alleviates their symptoms,

OPPOSITE PAGE: *A young girl demonstrates the ease of the Buteyko method.*

thus reducing dependency on drugs — but this of course is a gradual process that must be carefully monitored and controlled for the patient's safety. By following this careful health policy, in seven years of practice in Australia, the Buteyko clinics have helped all their patients in safety.

Choosing an Asthma Treatment

When investigating any natural approach to treating disease, the investigator must assess the method according to certain principles. The questions that an investigator asks are:

1. Does it fit with the principle of *primum non nocere* (First do no harm)?

The Buteyko method is simply a breathing technique, which involves no apparatus (except a stop watch!), no medication, no special environment, and no unnatural conditions or movements for the body to adapt to. It is natural and harmless. Not only does it do no harm, but people with many conditions positively benefit from it, not just asthmatics — because according to the Buteyko theory, not only do all asthmatics hyperventilate, but

This chapter is to familiarise the reader with the Buteyko method, and is not an instruction manual.

90% of the average population actually hyperventilate, and therefore risk hidden, long-term consequences.

Asthma

Professor Buteyko's Russian results showed that most patients with asthma achieved 90% alleviation of their symptoms and, with perseverance, the difficult last 10% of a patient's performance could be improved. The first closed clinical trial of the Buteyko treatment in Australia showed that, in mild to moderately severe asthma, patients achieved a 90% reduction in bronchodilator use over six weeks.

Sinusitis

Sinusitis has also been shown to improve with the Buteyko method, providing there is no severe nasal fracture, septum deviation or foreign body present in the nasal passages.

Hay Fever

Allergic rhinitis or hay fever is considered by Professor Buteyko to be asthma of the nose. The features are: congestion and mucosal swelling (similar to that in the lungs); thin mucus production with plasma leaking from inflamed blood vessels; and thick mucus. Unlike the situ-

The Buteyko method must not be learned without expert supervision. Consult your Buteyko teacher and your Medical Practitioner on any treatment for your health.

ation with muscles around the bronchial tubes in asthma, however, constriction of nasal muscles does not occur. Hay fever can be improved with the Buteyko method.

Sleep apnoea and snoring

Sleep apnoea (choking in one's sleep) and snoring can be controlled with perseverance, as will be seen in the next chapter.

Emphysema

This is a respiratory disease involving destroyed lung tissue, usually from smoking. Those with emphysema need more continuous application to the method, but even after one week of classes at a clinic people usually register enough improvement to encourage further practice.

No one who follows the technique to remedy a condition gets worse as a consequence, in either the short or long term.

Despite this, there were many early criticisms of the Buteyko method in Australia. A warning was once issued by the Victorian Branch of the Asthma Foundation, saying that the treatment was dangerous. Leaflets were distributed making this claim. Certain specialists hypothesised about a 'placebo effect' that would eventually dissipate,

This chapter is to familiarise the reader with the Buteyko method, and is not an instruction manual.

leaving patients just where they were before they learned the technique. Others warned about a 'honeymoon effect' that would wear off, and claimed that patients would actually deteriorate from that point. Practical experience with the Buteyko method has shown that these claims are unfounded.

2. Does this method use any drugs or medication?

The Buteyko technique uses no new drugs. However, all patients must bring all their medication to each class.

3. Can sufferers reduce their drug use?

Reduction of drugs or withdrawal is carried out gradually and responsibly under the guidance of a specially trained teacher and, often, the patient's doctor. If the patient's doctor has had no experience with the method, the Buteyko supervising medical officer is available for advice. Also the Buteyko workshops practise the open door policy with doctors, naturopaths and health practitioners. They are always welcome free of charge to attend alone or with their patients. Parents and relatives also attend at no extra charge. On two or three occasions, Professor Buteyko has been consulted by telephone in Moscow for advice when extreme cases presented themselves (see

> *The Buteyko method must not be learned without expert supervision. Consult your Buteyko teacher and your Medical Practitioner on any treatment for your health.*

next chapter). It is not only general practitioners who recommend patients to Buteyko clinics: respiratory physicians are on record as having found that patients improved after the practice of the method and have referred on other patients in consequence. The Asthma Foundations in Australia have also been known to give the Buteyko phone numbers to patients inquiring about the method.

4. How long does the treatment take?

The course consists of five to ten sessions of tuition. The sessions vary from one to two hours each. Usually five to seven sessions of one hour are enough for the patient to witness improvement and have confidence in the technique. However, the most severe cases, such as those who need regular hospital admittance, may require up to nine months of practice, to achieve the desired level of health.

5. What is the technique?

Patients are taught to normalise their breathing.

As we have seen, Professor Buteyko has investigated breathing patterns and made a study of over-breathing. He is convinced that over-breathing (hyperventilation) is the underlying cause of asthma and many other disor-

---

This chapter is to familiarise the reader with the Buteyko method, and is not an instruction manual.

---

ders. When a patient breathes less, and breathes more shallowly, a sequence of events occurs, due to a change in the relative levels of oxygen and carbon dioxide in the lungs and the blood stream. This leads to a more efficient oxygenation of the tissues of the body (see the next chapter for physiological details).Patients are asked to:

a) Breathe in and out, both through the nose only, to reduce breathing.

b) Tape the mouth up while sleeping unless there is some severe nasal condition. Adults can easily adapt to this but it often frightens parents initially — however, I have seen no child come to any harm over five years of recommending the practice. Partial taping can be practised initially until children and parents become more confident. A very light easily removable micropore tape is used.

c) Sleep on the left side and to avoid sleeping on the back. Sleeping on the back causes the most hyperventilation. Professor Buteyko's research has shown that sleeping on the left side causes least hyperventilation.

d) Increase the control pause and the maximum pause, which are defined next.

> *The Buteyko method must not be learned without expert supervision. Consult your Buteyko teacher and your Medical Practitioner on any treatment for your health.*

The Control Pause

The control pause is described as the time it takes someone to breathe out normally, then hold his or her breath in the out position until the *very first signs* of discomfort occur. That measurement is recorded, then the person continues to breathe through the nose in a shallow pattern. Most people can achieve 10 to 20 seconds, at rest. *Some cannot achieve even one second*, while others can do 40 seconds plus, quite naturally.

The idea is to succeed in holding the breath in the out position for up to 50 to 60 seconds to achieve the desired improvement. This is the measure of success.

The Maximum Pause

The maximum pause is the time it takes a person to breathe out normally, hold his or her breath in the out position and, through specially taught exercises and distractions, prolong this pause to the maximum time. With exercise, repetition and perseverance, some people surprise themselves with times of up to two minutes and even longer.

> *This chapter is to familiarise the reader with the Buteyko method, and is not an instruction manual.*

Patients are asked to come to classes for education and encouragement in these breathing exercises and to discuss problems and incidentals such as coincidental viruses, personal problems and so on.

Often, family members are invited to attend, free of charge, to further encourage the patients.

Between the classes, patients are urged to follow the rules (a) to (d) set out above (only nasal breathing, sleeping on left side etc.) and to follow a rigid regime of breathing exercises. Twice daily exercises for 20 minutes are required. Some people with mild illness stop their exercises after some two months and find their breathing has changed to a more shallow pattern. They can then stop their exercises altogether, as they no longer hyperventilate.

How Long Does One Practise the Technique?

Mild Cases

Mild cases of asthma tend to be episodic, and may be triggered by types of exercise or by viral infections. Once the Buteyko method has been learned and practised cor-

> *The Buteyko method must not be learned without expert supervision. Consult your Buteyko teacher and your Medical Practitioner on any treatment for your health.*

rectly, mild cases tend to need only episodic treatment with bronchodilators, and episodic breathing exercises.

Moderate Cases
Moderate cases are those who suffer from frequent asthma, or mild continuous asthma, and those who make regular use of a bronchodilator, with usually a steroid preventive inhaler. The exercise requirements for these people are two to four times per day for 20 minutes.

Severe Cases
Severe cases are usually on medication of two different types of bronchodilator inhalers plus steroid inhaler, with or without oral steroids and with or without other agents like methotrexate. They tend to need frequent hospital visits. The breathing exercises for people who suffer serious attacks, with protracted stays in hospital, are: three to five times per day for 20 to 30 minutes initially, later easing to two sessions. To achieve best results, these sufferers may take three to twelve months of practice.

This chapter is to familiarise the reader with the Buteyko method, and is not an instruction manual.

The Method of Prolonging Maximum Pause

First, the patient, under supervision, breathes out to the maximum and holds the nose and firmly closes the mouth while seated upright. Then, he/she holds the breath in expiration (that is, with 'empty' lungs) until he/she feels uncomfortable. The person then continues in expiration while utilising one or more distractions:

1) Body gyrations. These involve moving the torso about while holding the nose; flinging the body from side to side; putting the head between the knees; rocking from side to side; rocking forward and back.

2) Mobile exercises. Finally, the sitting gyrations don't distract the person enough and he/she stands up while holding the nose and begins to walk around the room in circles. He/she may walk outside the room, keeping on the move until he/she can really no longer hold the breath. In our clinic, this is often called the Groucho Marx walk.

3) Then, the person tries to prevent over-breathing by breathing strictly through the nose. He/she sits down again, and deliberately tries to achieve a shallow breathing

The Buteyko method must not be learned without expert supervision. Consult your Buteyko teacher and your Medical Practitioner on any treatment for your health.

39

equilibrium. After a rest of two to three minutes of shallow nose breathing, another control pause is carried out.

4) Children usually make a game of the exercises. When they start to have difficulty holding the breath, and really want to breathe in while they are sitting down and holding the nose, they pace out steps around the room and count up the number of steps in their heads. Some do squats, some jump up and down on the spot. Afterwards they compare their results with others. Both children and adults can be fiercely competitive over their achievements!

Adult asthma sufferers are usually accustomed to using peak flow meters. Rather than using the meters (which can, however, be used if desired), Buteyko practitioners prefer to use a single instrument — the stop watch. Success is measured as each person's increase in control pause is accurately timed.

Maximum pause can be stretched to surprising lengths but it is the *control pause* which is the final measure of success. If the feeling of first difficulty does not arise until 40 to 60 seconds have passed, a patient can feel confident that his/her respiratory problems are improving rapidly, that the hyperventilation is being corrected and that the oxygen and carbon dioxide ratio has been normalised.

> *This chapter is to familiarise the reader with the Buteyko method, and is not an instruction manual.*

A typical session of Buteyko breathing exercises

1. Take the pulse.

2. Control pause.

3. 3 minutes' shallow breathing

4. Maximum pause.

5. 3 minutes' shallow breathing

6. Control pause.

7. 3 minutes' shallow breathing

8. Control pause.

9. 3 minutes' shallow breathing

10. Maximum pause.

11. 3 minutes' shallow breathing

12. Control pause.

13. 3 minutes' shallow breathing

14. Take the pulse again.

The Buteyko method must not be learned without expert supervision. Consult your Buteyko teacher and your Medical Practitioner on any treatment for your health.

Control pause: The person takes a small breath in while sitting down, then breathes out and holds the breath until the first sign of discomfort (nose should be held during the control pause).

Maximum pause: The person takes a small breath in while sitting down, then breathes out and holds the breath for as long as possible. The person can try to distract him/herself by rocking back and forth in the chair and then by walking around.

Shallow breathing: The act of taking in less air. Initially the person feels as if he/she is not taking in enough air.

The pictures on pages 49–56 in the next chapter show asthma sufferers practising the method, including the control pause and the maximum pause.

Remember that if a person has a control pause of 15 seconds, he or she is breathing a volume of air per minute that is enough for four people. A control pause of 30 sec-

This chapter is to familiarise the reader with the Buteyko method, and is not an instruction manual.

Aims:

- To learn to shallow-breathe (i.e. take in less air, or take smaller breaths).

- To lengthen the control pause.

- To lengthen maximum pause and to use it instead of a bronchodilator. If the person feels an attack coming on, he/she can do one maximum pause, then 3 minutes' shallow breathing, then one more maximum pause. If no relief is felt, the patient can take one puff of the bronchodilator and if necessary one puff 5 minutes later.

onds indicates the person is breathing for two people. A control pause of 60 seconds means breathing is under control and he or she is breathing for one person.

The Buteyko method must not be learned without expert supervision. Consult your Buteyko teacher and your Medical Practitioner on any treatment for your health.

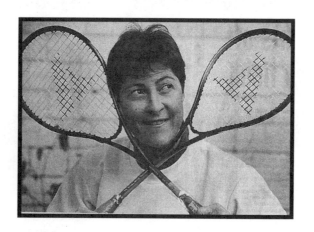

A New Lease of Life

Former Asthma Sufferers Tell Their Stories

I find that as a medical practitioner, nothing impresses me more than favourable reports coming from patients themselves. One favourable report is interesting, a few such reports impressive, but when one receives hundreds of favourable reports, the inherent scepticism in a scientific mind begins to dwindle and an avid interest emerges.

Fortunately, the first scientific clinical trial in the Western world carried out in Australia by the Asthma Foundation and the Buteyko team in 1995 showed, clearly and without prejudice, the real assistance that Buteyko offers to asthma sufferers.

On top of this, the words of improved and relieved patients speak volumes, and cannot be ignored. I have collected them here with the idea of showing not only how asthma can be controlled by proper breathing, but how other conditions also seem to be related to over-breathing, to the extent that when Buteyko practises are applied to these, they appear to be controllable in the same way that asthma can be.

The stories included here deal with a range of ages and

personalities, and throw light on many things — the way health information travels in our society, the concept of what is acceptable and unacceptable to us in our treatment of health problems, and what asthma and related diseases have traditionally cost so many people, in terms of illness, anxiety and in money. It is inspiring to read these stories and to see how people have improved their health and their lives.

Sufferers of Mild Asthma

Mild asthma is defined as episodic mild attacks of wheezing, occurring only occasionally and precipitated by allergy, irritants, cold air, exercise or emotion. These episodes can be of up to two weeks' duration, and occur more than six to eight weeks apart.

These attacks are easily alleviated by bronchodilators and the mild preventatives Intal or Tilade. A preventative is a drug prescribed to relieve the inflammation that can be casued by the use of a bronchodilator. However, a directive in 1997 from local and especially overseas respiratory specialists advised the early use of inhaled cortisone sprays (stronger preventatives) as well as bronchodilators, even in mild cases. Thus it is likely that people who suffer from mild asthma are therefore going to have stronger medication recommended to them in the future, unless current medical practice changes with reference to asthma medication.

KELLY

Kelly, aged 32, has a mild form of asthma. Her attacks began when she was 11 and had improved by the age of 20, but deteriorated again in her early thirties. Kelly is a jazzercise instructor, and found she needed to take two puffs of her Ventolin an hour before each class. She took three classes per week on average. Apart from this there were times when she would wheeze at night, her chest would feel tight and she would gasp for air.

She decided to attend a Buteyko clinic, and after the second Buteyko evening, she had a dramatic improvement. She is now off all medication and the jazzercise no longer stimulates her asthma attacks.

CATHERINE

Catherine is a mild asthmatic who does karate. This is her story, in her own words.

⭐ *There is light at the end of the tunnel for asthmatics! Constant wheezing, someone choking you, an elephant sitting on your chest ... sound familiar? About three years ago I developed asthma. I was given two turbuhalers of medication and sent on my way. Nothing much was explained about it except that I would have it for the rest of my life.*

This didn't quite agree with me, as I enjoyed my sport and didn't want it hindered in any way. So eventually I succumbed to taking daily medication, and I put up with the shaking and heart palpitations and God knows what else it was doing to my body.

Then on a regular visit to a specialist medical centre I was told about the Buteyko method, used to help asthmatics reduce their medication intake drastically, sometimes totally. This interested me a lot, especially as I had taken up karate and was exercising sometimes up to twice a day, which meant that I took 3000 mcg of corti-steroids a day [by puffer] for my asthma.

My first lesson with the Buteyko instructor was rather interesting. He explained that asthmatics breathe more than what they should. In fact I breathed five times more than necessary. Professor Buteyko believes that when we over-breathe we are breathing off too much carbon dioxide, so our body tries to stop this from happening and in defence narrows the airways so that the CO_2 stays in the body. This is all too much for one to believe, but as soon as the course starts you can feel the difference.

So, what I had to do was practise holding my breath, so as to retain CO_2. At first I accomplished a big 20 seconds [control pause]! I was surprised to find out that an average person should do 60 seconds. Then I had to practise 10 minutes of shallow breathing. This is harder than it sounds. My mouth was to be kept closed all the time (for those who know me that is a feat in itself). Breathing had to be really quiet and relaxed. It took a lot of concentration, you had to overcome this feeling of having lack of air. Eventually I got to 87 seconds and was then practising holding my breath while walking.

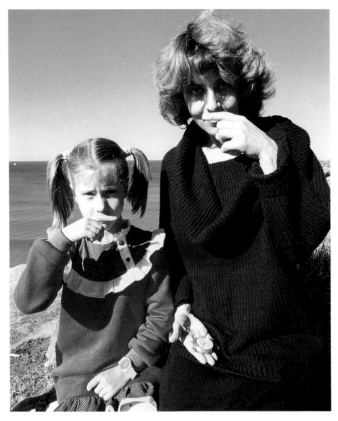

One way to normalise breathing is for a person to make sure he or she always breathes through the nose. Here, two patients practise shallow breathing, which is one of the Buteyko exercises. By holding a finger under the nose they can feel how much air they inhale and breathe out.

The Buteyko method must not be learned without expert supervision. Consult your Buteyko teacher and your Medical Practitioner on any treatment for your health.

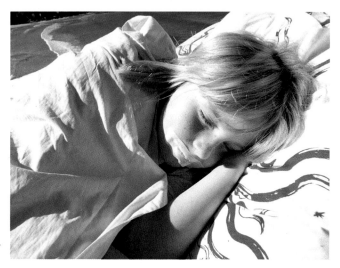

One can normalise breathing when asleep by breathing through the nose, and lying on the left side. Here, a patient demonstrates the practice of taping up the mouth, to promote nasal breathing while asleep. Strange though it looks at first, children and adults adapt well to this practice, which not only helps asthma sufferers but controls snoring (parents should not tape up the mouths of babies or small children, however). Partial taping can be practised at first with older children and adults. Practitioners advise the use of micropore tape, available from chemists, which pulls off easily and causes no allergy.

These pages are to familiarise the reader with the Buteyko method, and are not an instruction manual.

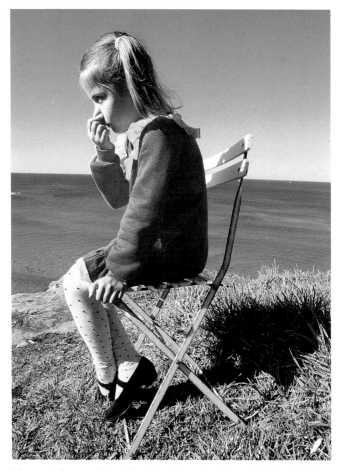

The control pause. The patient breathes out while seated, then holds the breath in the 'out' position until the first sign of discomfort occurs.

The Buteyko method must not be learned without expert supervision. Consult your Buteyko teacher and your Medical Practitioner on any treatment for your health.

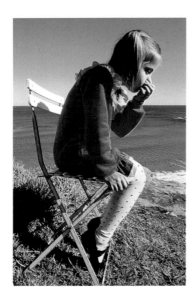

Prolonging the maximum pause by rocking forward and back, and flinging the body from side to side.

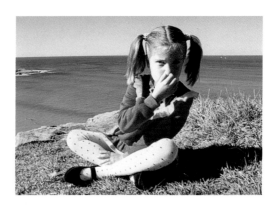

These pages are to familiarise the reader with the Buteyko method, and are not an instruction manual.

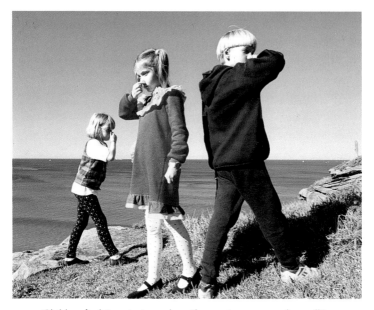

Children find it easier to prolong the maximum pause by walking around and counting steps in their heads.

The Buteyko method must not be learned without expert supervision. Consult your Buteyko teacher and your Medical Practitioner on any treatment for your health.

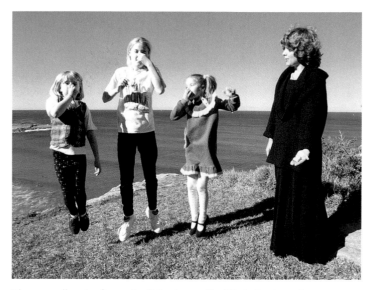

There are all sorts of ways to distract oneself while trying to prolong the maximum pause. Children especially enjoy jumping up and down on the spot.

These pages are to familiarise the reader with the Buteyko method, and are not an instruction manual.

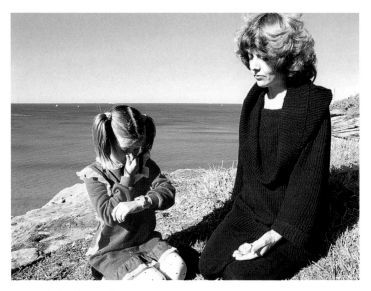

Timing the maximum pause.

The Buteyko method must not be learned without expert supervision. Consult your Buteyko teacher and your Medical Practitioner on any treatment for your health.

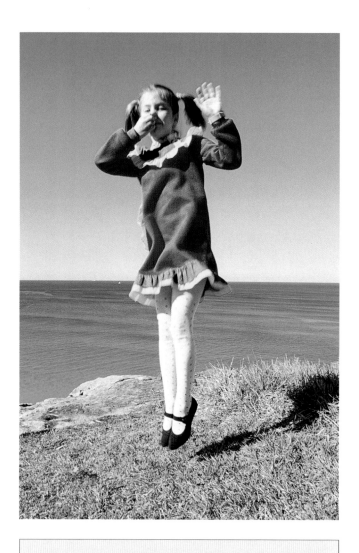

These pages are to familiarise the reader with the Buteyko method, and are not an instruction manual.

The next big feat was to accomplish exercise without medication. This can be quite scary if you have exercise-induced asthma. The instructor told me to practise my shallow breathing before the karate class for about half an hour, then if wheezing occurred during training to practise my breathing again for ten minutes. I also had to practise afterwards to return my breathing to normal.

Amazingly enough I didn't have any problems at all, In fact I found it easier to do the class. I wasn't breathing as heavily as I normally do, and didn't get as tired when I was sparring. One thing that was important was to keep my mouth closed while I was training (except when I Kiai, which means yelling while attacking).

Since I started the course I haven't needed to use my medication, even during a 3-hour training seminar on the weekend. It felt as though my lungs did not have anything to do with my exercising, and it was only my muscles that were taking part in the exercise — as though the only thing I had to do was the movement. I haven't had this feeling of freedom for the past three years!

VERA

Vera developed asthma as a baby in Russia, and this caused great anguish to the whole family. Her parents had a healthy lifestyle, ate healthy food, and preferred the natural approach to healing illness. So they were horrified to see their baby placed on bronchodilators, nebulisers and courses of antibiotics, and even courses of cortisone.

They tried alternatives like physiotherapy and different exercises, but the attacks continued. To begin with they did not go to a Buteyko clinic, as Vera was too young. However, when she was four-and-a-half they decided to book her into a clinic — only to discover that it was full for three months. Meanwhile they had decided to leave Russia with its harsh winters, and emigrate to Australia. They had already bought their tickets, and were afraid to change them and delay their flight. So they left Russia, terribly disappointed that they had not been able to give Vera the benefit of the method.

Ironically, after they boarded the flight they were told by a fellow passenger about the full effectiveness of Buteyko's therapy, which they believed Vera had missed out on. You can imagine their amazement when shortly after their arrival in Sydney they saw an advertisement for the Buteyko method. They wasted no time in taking Vera to a clinic. In four days she was off bronchodilators, and within two months she was off cortisone puffers. Five years later she uses Ventolin on one or two days per year if a virus irritates her airways. Vera is the delightful model on the cover of this book. Her mother was so impressed by her daughter's recovery that she became a Buteyko practitioner herself.

We have seen hundreds of patients like Kelly, Catherine and Vera who have mild asthma. Many tell me that they carried out the Buteyko exercises 'religiously' for two to three months but later lapsed. To their surprise, their asthma never returned, even years later, as their breathing had changed to a more shallow pattern. If a viral infection or severe stress causes a mild wheeze, a trained person can resume the exercises for a few days to achieve control or, if this fails, use a bronchodilator.

Sufferers of Moderate Asthma

If you have what is termed moderate asthma, it means you have more frequent attacks (closer than six to eight weeks apart) or chronic symptoms most days, requiring continuous bronchodilators and cortisone preventative at lower doses, and occasional outpatient hospital visits.

In moderate to severe asthma, Buteyko exercises need to be followed and continued more strictly. If a person decides to ease up on, or stop the exercises, symptoms can return. But these symptoms return slowly, gradually and safely. This usually means that the sufferer gradually restarts drug treatment — but there is a choice to return to the exercises, and if they are followed they remain effective.

ALAN

Alan, a moderately severe asthmatic, wrote this after attending his Buteyko sessions.

☆ *I have been a chronic asthmatic since 1984. As a 64-year-old, I was resigned to medication and limited activity* for the rest of my life. I may add I have spent many hours in hospitals due to severe asthma attacks. My nebuliser has been in use at least twice daily and I frequently also had to resort to my trusty puffer.

My condition was so bad, I had to retire from work in 1984 and my life assurance was also paid out.

Six weeks ago, friends recommended I go to a Buteyko workshop. I am aware of the short period since I first went to the workshop but I have not had any Ventolin since and only used my Pulmicort twice. To me, this is like getting a second chance at life. Last Sunday, I was able to wheel 21 barrow loads of bark around our gardens and despite sweating, had no adverse effects from the exercise I had not been able to enjoy for ten years.

I sincerely hope the NSW Asthmatic Foundation instigates and hastens investigations into the Buteyko breathing technique as I am convinced many asthmatics will gain much relief doing the exercises and thereby decreasing their medication [written prior to the Queensland scientific trial].

The amount of money saved by Medicare, hospitals and health departments must also benefit all Australians.

People like Alan who obtain such effective relief from Buteyko exercises find that if they are continued, there is no 'honeymoon period' that wanes, as predicted by sceptics — and there are no sudden deteriorations or surprises. Also, occasionally missing a day or two of exercise makes little difference.

If symptoms gradually return and you no longer want to practise the technique or would like to stop the exercises for a month or six weeks due to extraordinary time pressures, you can resume medication for as long as it takes, then practise the exercises again when you are able. Jane, whose story follows, is a case in point.

JANE

Jane, aged 36, is a former patient who rang me one day with an unusual request for advice. She had had brilliant success with the Buteyko breathing method and was off all treatment for one year, but her workload was about to increase dramatically for six weeks and she was afraid she might not be able to do any exercises for that period.

Strictly for the convenience of it, she wanted to use the puffers for the six weeks, and once the frantic period was over, she intended to resume exercise and reduce the puffers as she had done previously.

I prescribed Ventolin and Pulmicort, her previous medication over one year prior, and said she could gradually start taking them if the asthma symptoms returned. She found the symptoms did return, but slowly over two to three weeks, even though she had been a moderate asthmatic and was frantically busy and stressed, as she predicted.

Even after five weeks and stressed to the limit, she never used as much medication as before learning the breathing method.

When the busy time had passed, she easily resumed the exercises and once again became medication free.

I would like to add that most people would have intensified or continued their practice of the exercises in the above situation instead of resorting to the drugs, but this is a good illustration that one always has a choice. Her case history demonstrates the flexibility and the safety of the method.

LOLA

Like Alan, Lola is in her early sixties. She tells her own interesting story.

☆ *Up until now, over 15 years, I have tried everything conceivable to help my asthma, at times working an extra job to pay for some relief, or cure, e.g. acupuncture, iridology, herbalist, wholistic clinics etc. No relief, never mind any cure.*

I was very sceptical when I heard of the Buteyko course and after hearing the Asthma Foundation on the Mike Gibson show I put it out of my mind, until the next evening during a severe attack while wondering if I could take the nebuliser mask off long enough to ring an ambulance.

I thought, if I live through this one, I'll give the treatment a go. I'll try something just one more time. I have, at times during severe attacks, thought of self-euthanasia, too tired to drag myself off to work any more. My doctor had suggested many years ago to go on a sickness pension, but I love to work.

So, with a sceptical mind and the money that was to do the rust on the car, I joined. Believe me it's the best thing that has happened to me in 15 years and I am so happy that I decided to let the rust go. I can work longer hours now anyway and save up to have the car done.

I was on 300 mg Theodur am and pm, puffer or nebuliser every 2 hours, followed by Becloforte and oral steroids. I am now on one puff Ventolin am and pm, followed by Becloforte. I always carry my puffer with me, as we are told in class to always keep our medication close by.

I am not cured, but I can control the asthma attacks. I'm sleeping well and am calm and relaxed. My workmates are surprised at the different me, because they laughed when I said I was going to do the course and said I would fall for the four-card trick.

I ate beetroot in vinegar a little while ago, which is bad for me, and I started to wheeze. I did my correct breathing, and the wheeze was gone in two minutes.

Yesterday, I was feeling down for reasons other than my asthma, and I just had to have some chocolate. I actually ate a whole block of Toblerone, which was suicidal in my previous condition. Not a thing happened. Not even a wheeze. I just can't believe it. Soon, I am going to try some pizza, for the first time in 15 years. This is the best $400 I have ever spent.

I am writing to the head of the Asthma Foundation to beg him to look into this course so all the other asthmatics may be helped.

DOMINIC

David, the father of six children including Dominic, is a so-licitor in his early fifties. All his children were raised on natural foods according to natural health guidelines. He was proud of the fact they were all healthy. The only thing he could not achieve was a natural way to relieve his son's asthma.

Dominic was nine years old when he first went to a Buteyko clinic. He had suffered from asthma for his whole life, and had been attended to by asthma specialists, none of whom suggested the Buteyko treatment.

After only one week of doing the exercises, Dominic's asthma was under control.

Knowing that 800 people plus died from asthma in Australia annually, David immediately decided he wanted to spread the word. His message is summarised from the *Natural Health Society Magazine* of April/May 1995.

☆ *'These deaths are unnecessary. The medical profession must wake up and forget medicine and treat the cause like Buteyko does. It's long overdue to stop seeking more and more medicines to alleviate the symptoms and instead treat the cause.*

'There are apparently one million people in Australia who suffer from asthma. If they can all cure themselves, it will be a great saving for the public purse.'

Why is there no official approbation for a method which is extremely effective in treating a whole range of related dis-

orders such as allergies, rhinitis, sleeping disorders, breath-ing problems, hypertension and angina?

David says: 'If it takes ten years before the Buteyko sys-tem is given official government approbation and funding, that translates into 8000 unnecessary deaths. That is a lot of heartache which can be avoided. If the Russian govern-ment fully endorses the "Buteyko Method" then so should ours, and the sooner the better.'

ANNE

Anne is a young flight attendant in her early twenties. She had a past history of moderate asthma and severe si-nusitis for ten years. Family history often reveals a ten-dency to asthma that is inherited, but with Anna the only other person who suffered from asthma was her niece, who had asthma at six months. Anna's allergies were dust mite, moulds and salicylates.

Anne is an example of someone with a cluster of con-ditions that all came from the same cause, though she was unaware of this for many years. Meanwhile she had to cope with daily life and her job. Her treatment con-sisted of:

- Ventolin, two puffs twice daily
- Becloforte, one puff twice daily
- Two courses of reducing doses of oral Prednisone

Complementary treatment:
- Vitamin C oral, I g daily, later increased
  to 2 g daily
- Sambuccus complex (herbals for sinus
  by Blackmore)
- Garlic

She was plagued by an intermittent blocked right ear, sinusitis and asthma. Her work subjected her to air conditioning, temperature changes, anti-mosquito and insect sprays and pressure changes (more painful in her right ear than her left, and in her sinuses). She also had a fluid sensation in her right ear. Her right ear was at times oversensitive to the radio and telephone and at other times, she found it hard of hearing. Also, on take off and landing, she experienced severe pain in her right ear. This made her work as a flight attendant almost unbearable.

Treatment for three months of one year:

April 10   Middle ear infection treated by local medical officer with Ceclor 250 mg three times daily for five days.

April 15   Referred to Ear, Nose and Throat specialist who diagnosed chronic rhinitis with intermittent blocking of the eustachian tube by a nasal polyp. Treated with Rhinocort (cortisone nasal spray) twice daily to each nostril for three weeks.

(At this stage, Anne was thus on two types of cortisone spray, nasal and lung.)

April 19   C.A.T. scan (special X-ray) ordered.

May 9   Chronic low-grade infection. Throat swab negative.

May 27   Head cold. Sinus infection.

May 30   Laryngitis. Prescribed Augmentin (double antibiotic) 250 mg three times daily.

June 4   Vibramycin 100 mg daily for seven days.

June 15   Specialist C.A.T. scan carried out.

June 17   Buteyko course commenced.

June 21   Specialist prescribes Vibramycin.

June 23   Extreme paranasal sinusitis. Prescribed Rhinocort. C.A.T. scan results come in, confirming blocked sinuses.

June 27   On continuing practice of her Buteyko method a coral-like structure drops out from high in her throat on the right side.

This coral-like blockage was thought to be hardened mucus expelled from the right eustachian tube. All discomfort disappeared soon after this and the ear was no longer blocked. Anne's sinuses improved. Only a slight irritation remained in the throat. This was thought to be candida due to the Rhinocort spray and antibiotics. Upon stopping the Rhinocort and all antibiotics, Anne found that her throat rapidly improved and she has remained well on no drug treatment for her throat and nose, with only the Buteyko breathing exercises adhered to.

It took Anne six months before she could safely and comfortably stop all treatment for her asthma as well. The last medication to go was the Becloforte. She has continued her strenuous work as a flight attendant.

JOAN AND HER HUSBAND

Joan's case is fascinating: she first learned of the Buteyko method after she and her husband had sought a wide range of help and paid out a great deal of money to deal with her husband's health problems, which included snoring, sleep apnoea (choking while asleep), and physical collapses as a result. Joan also suffered from asthma and angina, but the care and time spent on her husband's ailments took first place in her mind.

When you read her letter to a specialist, you will understand the terrible disruption illness can cause in people's lives, and how frantic they can be to find a cure — to the extent of considering the purchase of extremely expensive equipment.

You will see how Joan at first observed her husband's progress with his sleep apnoea (choking while asleep) and then applied the method to her asthma and angina.

☆ *I was interested to hear your [a respiratory specialist's] remarks at the Asthma Foundation's Conference in October 1995 about people who take the risk of pursuing non-traditional paths to regain their health. Since you retain an 'open mind' on the subject, I am taking the trouble to give you the benefit of 13 years of observations.*

For all this time, except for the last year, my husband disturbed my sleep with his cacophony of sounds. But these problems pre-date me. My step-children who are now in their mid '20s remember, from a young age, being given the task of pulling his hair to keep him awake when on weekend drives.

Last year, we were living in Darwin and he was adversely affected by the heat, a very stressful job and up to three 14-hour plane trips per month. Although our diet did not change nor his drinking habits, he increased his weight from 80 to 90 kg and showed signs of jaundice. He also experienced two very nasty 'turns' in the night involving bouts of diarrhoea and nausea. Apparently, he had had three other similar 'collapses' in the preceding 20 years. In the fourth of these, he fainted in a toilet in Darwin. The fifth extreme episode occurred in Canberra while he was assigned to a senior position. The GP he visited dismissed the episode as food poisoning (although the family all had the same to eat). He was referred to the local sleep clinic in response to his request for information on laser surgery to 'cure' snoring.

The findings [which Joan attached to her letter]: a diagnosis of moderate Sleep Apnoea and a recommendation to get hooked up to a CPAP machine at night, for life (cost $1500+). That diagnosis cost $585. After diligent inquiry by a family friend in Sydney, my husband postponed the second all-night appointment at the sleep clinic for the machine, to keep an appointment in Bankstown on 18/10/94 with Australia's leading specialist in laser surgery. Dr B's counsel was not encouraging:

• most of his patients undergo surgery [laser surgery that removes tissue from inside the throat] because their spouses find the noise of the CPAP machine more disruptive than the natural snoring,
• in almost half the cases, surgery will be required again in a few years to remove 'regrowth',
• my husband would be in too much pain to work, for up to three weeks,
• by nasendoscopy examination, he deduced my husband's windpipe collapses to 15% of its normal diameter (which creates the obstruction) — laser surgery could not do anything about this but might help with the snoring,
• the specialist discouraged my husband from making a booking for surgery until after he had thought about it in view of the 60% probability that no benefit would result even in the short term.

We duly paid the $154.40 fee but so far have not incurred the expense of the operation.

Perhaps you can imagine that this conflicting advice from two of your eminent, specialist colleagues left us in a quandary. Having diligently pursued the conventional route, we were left wondering what to do. Fortuitously, we stumbled across an advertisement in the Canberra Times by your research colleague, a local physiotherapist and Buteyko practitioner. The small advertisement caught our attention because my first father-in-law had told me last year that after 65 years of asthma, he had finally found relief by daily adherence to this new regime. Mention was made in the advertisement of its efficacy in the treatment of snoring and sleep apnoea (and other breathing disorders).

We were not able to follow up because of our return to Darwin but a few days later the NT News carried a story about a local child's breakthrough with asthma. The Perth-based practitioner accepted a booking and $450 for his next five-day workshop in Darwin, which began on the first of November, 1994.

I remain amazed by the fact that my husband has not snored since. Nor does he have to be kept awake while driving (or in meetings after lunch). He also now fits into the suits we bought in London while working there (1988–1992). This loss in weight did not result from a change in our diet but only in his breathing.

Like you, my husband seeks objective explanations and evidence for such phenomena, so we spent another $585 (including $441.30 from Medicare) at the sleep clinic on 1/6/95 (exactly six months after commencing the Buteyko course). These results [attached to Joan's letter] indicate he has normal sleep architecture. The local specialist attributes this to weight loss which he recorded as 6 kg, although as attested to by my husband's London suits, he used to snore whatever he weighed.

Before the second sleep-over, my husband tried without success to get a 'minute volume' test at our local hospital. The specialist there and the diagnoser are both disparaging of the test on the grounds that people can control and influence their breathing rates. Undeterred in his search for objective data, he travelled to Brisbane on 4 May, 1995, and the results are enclosed. As we understand it, his figures are still above normal levels (4.5 L/min). Unfortunately we have no baseline to compare with because (surprisingly) your colleagues don't seem to consider hyperventilation as a factor in respiratory 'disorders'. What I do know is:

• in former times, after being banished one night from our bed in Darwin for a particularly orchestral performance, my husband speculated the next morning that he 'breathed too much',
• independent observers such as his work colleagues who deal with him by phone have commented on the change in his breathing patterns. His colleagues who work in the same office are amazed by his increased vitality and improved appearance,
• he no longer stops breathing while awake and then resumes with a 'sigh'.

In the light of this exposure to my husband's conditions, it came as a shock to hear you discount the advertisements for the Buteyko method and its claimed efficacy for sleep apnoea.

Your general 'tone' regarding patients who explore health options not (yet) accepted by the traditionalists, was of concern to me.

My retired father-in-law was the Chief (Electrical) Engineer for the Sydney County Council, my husband has an honours degree and I also graduated from Sydney University. We do not follow whims. Nor do we waste our money. We (and the tax payers) have spent on conventional diagnosis, $1,317.40 — which is significantly more than on the Buteyko Method ($450). The very hefty costs of the CPAP machine ($1,250–$1,600) and/or laser surgery have proved unnecessary.

Incidentally, I have not attended the Buteyko course. However, I suffered asthma during my first marriage. Stress associated with everyday family life triggered very severe chest pains. My husband's Buteyko practitioner from Perth suggested that my symptoms could be caused by hyperventilation.

This made some sense since all the doctors I have consulted failed to establish any other cause. By applying the simplest of the Buteyko techniques, I avoided full onset of these excruciating pains. Buoyed by this evidence, I have worked quietly on applying the reduced breathing techniques. There is still plenty of stress in my life but now I get neither asthma nor chest pains. Some friends who suffer from hay fever, particularly in November, also find my advice stops their attacks.

If you think I am on the wrong path, please drop me a line to put me right.

Health revolution

Breath of life

WHEN Julie Lobel was five years old she was one of the first children in Australia to be put on Ventalin spray. Since then she has battled severe asthma. She had collapsed lungs as a child and has lost count of the times she almost died after being admitted to hospital with asthma. Later in life, she became dependant on steroid-based medication which gave her mood swings, weight gain and bouts of laryngitis every six weeks.

However, since learning a simple breathing system called the Buteyko method, she has not had an asthma attack, no longer relies on Ventalin and is cutting down on steroid drugs.

"Last year I had a very bad bout of asthma. I couldn't walk from my bedroom to the bathroom without having an attack," says Ms Lobel, who is now 30. I was admitted to hospital where they gave me a dose of an adrenaline drug. I was sent home on some adrenaline medication and thought I had better do something about this."

Soon after, she heard about Buteyko from a colleague. "Within a week, I was seeing results not only in my breathing but my laryngitis cleared up. I had a lot of hayfever, which cleared up as did the mucus and the sneezing – I used to sneeze all day.

"Because my sleep was disturbed, I would wake up feeling tired no matter how much sleep I had had. Now I have five hours sleep a night and I feel great."

The most dramatic part of the treatment was sleeping for three weeks with her mouth taped to train her body to breathe through the nose.

Thanks to this and some simple breathing exercises, Ms Lobel is now able to renovate her Canberra house

Relief for a patient who was happy to put her drug puffer 'under wraps': part of an article from the Sun Herald of 13 April 1997

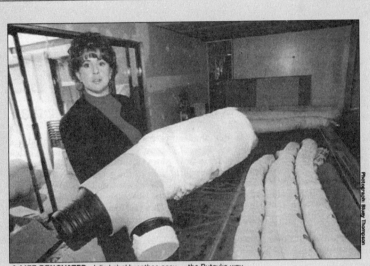

A LIFE RENOVATED: Julie Lobel breathes easy ... the Buteyko way.

Sufferers of Severe Asthma

Severe asthma means chronic, severe, continuous symptoms of wheeze and cough requiring maximum amounts of bronchodilators and cortisone preventatives and often oral cortisone courses and the addition of other medication. More frequent hospital outpatient visits and admissions are necessary and frequent night 'attacks' are features of severe asthma.

GIOVANNA

Giovanna, mother of Kelly mentioned among the mild asthma cases, developed asthma after suffering from cardiac congestion in 1983. She had been a heavy smoker until then. In 1989 she also developed sleep apnoea and was always feeling depressed. It would take her more than an hour to get out of bed each morning and she would be constantly drowsy. She and her husband were forced to move to a house with no stairs and no carpet, even though she had previously worked as a cleaner. She had been on maximal asthma treatment as well as maximum oral medication for heart failure.

Following her attendance at the Buteyko course with her daughter, Giovanna noticed an improvement almost immediately. She is now able to engage in physical activity and no longer requires any asthma-related medication. She has also experienced huge and continuing weight loss.

Many of my patients report that they have lost weight when their metabolism (chemical reactions in the body) normalises after the breathing course.

EMMA

Emma was diagnosed with asthma at the age of six. From then until she reached the age of eight, her condition got steadily worse, even though she followed a medication regime.

When she originally came to the Buteyko Clinic, her attacks were daily and very severe. Her medication regime was as follows:

- Ventolin 2.5 ml via nebuliser (mask-pump) four times daily
- Atrovent 2 ml via nebuliser four times daily
- Pulmicort 800 mcg daily
- Prednisone/Prednisolone (Corticosteroid) 10 mg daily

On commencement of the reconditioning of Emma's breathing pattern, a reduction in her symptoms occurred. After seven weeks, she no longer suffered any symptoms and this situation has continued to this day. Now she only takes Pulmicort if viruses are affecting her; the dose is 100 mcg twice daily at these times. Otherwise she takes no medication for asthma.

BARBARA

Barbara, aged 61, suffered from asthma for 49 years, from the age of 12. Prior to commencing the Buteyko course to recondition her breathing, Barbara's medication intake was as follows:

- Theo-dur 300 mg twice daily
- Bricanyl 500 mcg six puffs daily
- Atrovent six puffs daily
- Pulmicort 400 mcg six puffs daily
- She also regularly needed to take larger doses of Ventolin through her nebuliser (face-mask)

and courses of Prednisone/Prednisolone
(corticosteroid) — 25 mg.

Barbara worked extremely hard on normalising her breathing pattern. Her asthmatic symptoms reduced to the point that she was able to drop all of her medication except for her Pulmicort, which she has reduced to four puffs daily. She continues her exercise, hoping to improve completely.

CHRISTANA

Christana was diagnosed with asthma at four years of age. She was the only one in her immediate or extended family who suffered from asthma, except for her half brother, who had mild asthma. From the age of 13 onwards she was faced with a rapid deterioration of her condition. By the time she was 17 she and her parents had sought far and wide for help — she was attending a psychologist and a psychiatrist, as well as a respiratory specialist.

Despite her condition she had been an athlete in her earlier years, but now she found herself unable to do any sport. She could not attend school regularly, and her condition was so bad that at times she found it hard to walk across a room. She became so short of breath that she could not even sustain a simple telephone conversation. Christana says that at this time she used to put all her cortisone and other pills in a blender with juice, because she just could not swallow them all whole.

If Christana did manage to go out anywhere, she had to take her nebuliser and solutions with her, as she needed the nebuliser half-hourly day and night when awake. During the night she would have to wake up at least once every two or three hours. If she went longer than two hours without the nebuliser she usually needed admission to hospital, where she would be put on a drip. Asthma cut Christana off from her friends, her education, and a normal life. She felt absolutely without hope. The drugs she used:

- Nebulisers ½–2 hourly (Ventolin at 10 mg, Atrovent)
- Prednisone 50–100 mg daily
- Bricanyl infusion, through a syringe driver given subcutaneously. This is an English technique: 5 mg over 24 hours, later up to 20 mg over 24 hours (Intragan)
- Methotrexate 10 mg per week and increased to 15 mg per week.

Allergies: Christana was allergic to all the following: cats, dogs, dust, dust-mite, pollens, wheat, rice, cereals, lettuce, soy milk, apple, mould, dyes, sprays, alcohol, fish, pears, MSG, all nuts.

Course of Treatment: Christana travelled from her home in Tasmania to Sydney to try the Buteyko method. At first she was unable to do the method at all, as she had no pause, not even one second — she was hyperventilating continually. The following alternative treatments were instigated to complement her medical treatment.

Christana started on a course of IV (Intravenous) vitamin C 15 g, three times per week, vitamin B_{12} injection IV (given intramuscularly). She was admitted to hospital and given more than 1000 mg Hydrocortisone overnight during a severe attack, then discharged on the above treatment. Two or three times a week, she was given an antispasmodic, Mg So4 (magnesium sulphate) by intramuscular injection.

Then her new breathing regime began. Intensive shallow breathing was introduced frequently, to increase control and maximum pause. Christana's control pause was two seconds, her maximum pause three to four seconds. The Buteyko practice and alternative treatments started in April 1993. The Buteyko method usually involves five to seven one-hour sessions, but there was a much more difficult gravity of illness in this case, and Christana needed to persevere much longer.

She had five admissions to hospital during her time in Sydney. These hospital stays were brief, between one and two days. She saw a leading respiratory specialist and one allergy specialist in Sydney.

The Buteyko instructor also rang Professor Buteyko in Russia, for additional advice. On hearing of her treatment he said, 'She is obviously not absorbing Prednisone orally, so it must be given intravenously.' Professor Buteyko also suggested Christana would benefit from Kenacort IM, but in Australia Kenacort (Triamcinolone) is used mainly for arthritic inflammatory conditions and skin inflammatory conditions. As the medical supervisor while Christana was attending the clinic, I recommended that we use IV Hydrocortisone. Christana was given 50 mg intravenously by the doctor in the afternoon, then 25 mg IM by a trained nurse, administered six-hourly, totalling 125 mg. For the next month (June), Christana was given 100 mg IM daily, Monday to Friday, and over the last three weeks of her stay in Sydney, this was gradually reduced to 5 mg.

Christana continued her intensive shallow breathing exercises, and by November she was able to achieve a control pause of 21 seconds and a maximum pause of 60 seconds. *On New Year's Eve, she was completely off all treatment* — it had taken eight-and-a-half months of breathing training and gradual reduction of her drug therapy to achieve this, but she had done it.

To top this success, she had lost a phenomenal 15 kg in weight, due to the elimination of her cortisone intake.

The only deficit which remains for Christana, apart from the occasional need to use a nebuliser (about once a month) is osteoporosis, bone and musculoligamentous discomfort (muscle and tendon pain) that she suffers. These are all due to the chronic corticosteroids given for some years, which leached calcium from her bones. She is presently taking Rocaltrol (Calcitriol) twice daily in order to try to improve the bone density. She can now jog, swim and dance regularly and has trained to become a Buteyko Practitioner in Tasmania.

Caren wins fight for life

Squash champ KOs asthma

By NATALIE WILLIAMS

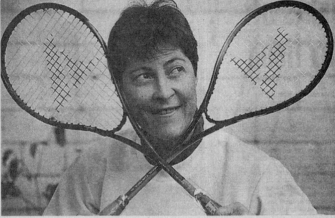

Confident: Former squash champion Caren Clonda is ready for her comeback

THE only Australian to win the British Junior Squash Championship is about to make a comeback to the courts after 15 years battling life-threatening asthma.

At 33, Caren Clonda is confident of returning to the professional circuit next year, bolstered by her faith in the controversial Buteyko Russian breathing technique.

A "natural" at squash from the age of 14, Caren was Australian and British Junior Champion in 1979 and six times NSW (Open) squash champion from 1981. She was ranked fifth in the world in 1983 and 1984 and third in Australia from 1983-85.

At her peak, Caren was training 4-5 hours a day doing weights, anaerobics, aerobics, sprintwork and playing squash.

But her professional career was ended by severe asthma and then Chronic Fatigue Syndrome, which she blames on the enormous amount of medication prescribed for her asthma.

Caren was so sick — "my immune system has had enough, it's suppressed and depressed" — she thought she would never walk onto a squash court again.

"Like everyone else, I was very sceptical about the Buteyko program, but I had tried hypnotherapy, counselling, acupuncture, past life regression — everything," she said at her Crows Nest home.

"Really, I tried it out of sheer desperation.

"In February (this year) my mother took me to a Buteyko lecture and I thought 'I've got nothing to lose, why not give it a go?'

"I haven't looked back and I describe Buteyko's work as the discovery of the century."

In 1952, Russian scientist and doctor Konstantin Buteyko discovered what he claims is the real cause of asthma — overbreathing, or hyperventilation.

Prof Buteyko's research has shown that this deep-overbreathing pattern can be the cause of a wide variety of problems including asthma, emphysema, sleep apnoea, allergies, sinusitis, migraines and high blood pressure.

He claims that symptoms of asthma and many other problems can be decreased simply by normalising a patient's breathing.

Caren said traditional treatments for asthma offered only temporary relief as they did not affect the real cause — overbreathing.

"Asthmatics breathe too much so, as a defence mechanism, the body signals the bronchial muscles to spasm, constricting the airflow to and in the lungs to stop this overbreathing," she said.

"The Buteyko technique teaches the asthmatic to reprogram their breathing pattern, enabling them to control their breathing.

"At first, this helps them overcome attacks, then in time and with practice they can actually prevent attacks."

Caren now has three aims — to stage a comeback next year, to make more people aware of the Buteyko breathing method and to press health departments and the ASMA Foundation to "open their minds" and research Prof Buteyko's claims.

A new lease of life for a former squash champion: an article from the Sunday Telegraph of 17 July 1994.

JOSHUA

By the time Joshua was 14 he had almost given up the will to live, he was so tired of always fighting for breath. He had been a severe asthmatic since the age of one — as long as he could remember. He had suffered respiratory arrest and been admitted to hospital many times — in just one year, he found himself in hospital 23 times. His medication included large doses of steroids and bronchial dilators — Oral Prednisone, Intal Forte, Ventolin, Atrovent.

Joshua's attacks affected every aspect of his life and meant that his daily activities, his schooling, his friendships, and normal childhood fun and games were desperately restricted. Not only did he have a disease to cope with, but the high doses of drugs he needed were also affecting his general health. His bones had become brittle and his weight ballooned as a result of the cortisone that he was prescribed.

Joshua came to a Buteyko clinic with this frightening history of severe, life-threatening asthma. After only six weeks of treatment, his condition improved dramatically. After a further few weeks, his chest was clear and he presently requires only the occasional puff of Ventolin.

Joshua's mother was amazed at the rapid effects of the breathing method. She noticed the improvement within only a few days, and reported: 'He was able to sleep through the night and could walk up stairs without becoming breathless.' Now, she has an overwhelming sense of relief and joy in what she has described as his

EVERY BREATH YOU TAKE

'miraculous' improvement. He has lost weight, is working part-time and is able to look to the future with optimism.

BERNARD

Bernard, who is in his mid-seventies, suffered from both asthma and emphysema when he saw a Buteyko practitioner. He attended a clinic, and later wrote this letter.

⭐ *Early in February this year, I made inquiries from you regarding the Buteyko method of Asthma control. At the time, you declined to give an opinion over the phone, even though you recommended the method to me, and asked me, should I attend the course, would I comment to you on the results. I have pleasure in so doing.*

Firstly, I am a 'late onset' asthmatic, aged 74, the asthma first becoming apparent in August, 1991. I also have emphysema. In 1992/3, I was hospitalised several times in Port Pirie General Hospital and attended by Dr G.P., my local physician. I also consulted a specialist on two occasions in Adelaide, Dr L. at her rooms in North Adelaide.

*While in hospital, I had medication as follows —
Nebuliser four times daily with Ventolin Nebules 5 mg and Atrovent 250 mcg. Also, Prednisolone with Peak Flow reading between 200–350 l/hr. After returning home on the last occasion, I was using the nebuliser with the same medication as before — four times daily — with six to eight puffs Pulmicort and depending on my condition, I was able*

to reduce the medication to a degree but I still used the nebuliser daily before retiring, with six to eight puffs Pulmicort daily. I also carried a Ventolin puffer in the form of Respolin with me at all times. I also considered it necessary to carry the nebuliser with me and if required, run it from the car battery.

My physical condition at the beginning of the year was, I felt, poor, in that I had great difficulty in walking more than 20 to 30 yards. I had to give up my favourite hobby, fishing, as I found it impossible to launch and retrieve the boat by myself. Gardening, also a hobby, had to be virtually stopped.

I attended the Buteyko course which began on 19 February and I must report the results have been truly amazing in that I now feel as well as I did prior to 1991. I am now able to resume my fishing and gardening interests and also am able to walk without stopping, recently covering approximately five km without a break.

My medication currently is two puffs of Pulmicort daily. I also carry a Respolin Auto haler with me but rarely find the necessity to use it. My nebuliser has not been used since the course began in February.

My doctor agrees that I have improved immensely and I feel sure he would agree with what I have told you, should you contact him.

Finally, I will be only too pleased to answer any question you may wish to ask, as I feel, having benefited so greatly myself, this method should be made easily available to all who require it.

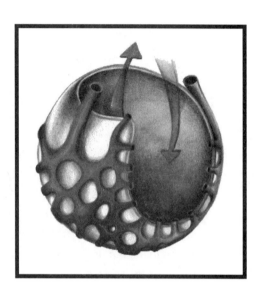

How Does the Buteyko Method Work?

The Physiology of Breathing

This chapter takes a close look at what we have already read about in the first chapter — Professor Konstantin Buteyko's beliefs about human over-breathing, and the effect it may have on our health.

We all know that breathing plays a vital role in the human organism. Nutrition is of major importance to us, yet we can survive without food for weeks, and without water for days. But if the average individual is without air for three to five minutes, he or she cannot survive. We normally breathe 20–30,000 times every 24 hours.

The Importance of Carbon Dioxide

The human breathing system developed in ancient geological times when carbon dioxide (CO_2) in the air and water was present in tens of per cent. It is probably due to this factor that a definite concentration of carbon dioxide — 7% approximately — is essential in each human cell

DIAGRAM A

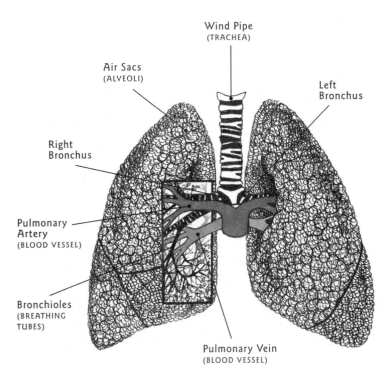

Wind Pipe
(TRACHEA)

Air Sacs
(ALVEOLI)

Left
Bronchus

Right
Bronchus

Pulmonary
Artery
(BLOOD VESSEL)

Bronchioles
(BREATHING
TUBES)

Pulmonary Vein
(BLOOD VESSEL)

This drawing shows the structure of the lungs and indicates the major blood vessels, airways, and air sacs.

to sustain normal life. The gaseous mix in the womb is an interesting indicator of the ideal human environment. Here, there exists between 7% to 8% of carbon dioxide.

Over the ages, the evolving human body has had to face a problem of the decrease in carbon dioxide in our air, from a level of more than 20% in ancient times to the current level of 0.03%. Human evolution has compensated for this by creating an internal air environment within the alveolar spaces (small air sacs) in the lungs. These alveoli normally contain around 6.5% of carbon dioxide.

The optimal level of carbon dioxide in the lung air sacs is around 6.5%. If for any reason (such as over-breathing) it falls below this, there is a gradual alkaline reaction in the lungs (called respiratory alkalosis). At the extreme, if the carbon dioxide level falls to below 3%, shifting the pH (the acidity level) to eight (more alkaline), the organism dies. When the carbon dioxide level is lowered, the gradual alkaline reaction in the lungs carries through to the blood, and total blood CO_2 will also be low. This decrease in total blood CO_2 is called alkalosis. The kidneys try to 'buffer' or correct this imbalance. This partially makes up for the CO_2 deficiency, but it sets up a course of events which change for the worse the rate and efficiency of activity of all the vitamin and enzyme systems in our body. And it is these systems that run our energy and vitality.

While air is held in the lungs, the molecules it contains pass through the walls of the alveoli and into the blood, to be carried around the system and nourish the

(continued on page 92)

DIAGRAM B

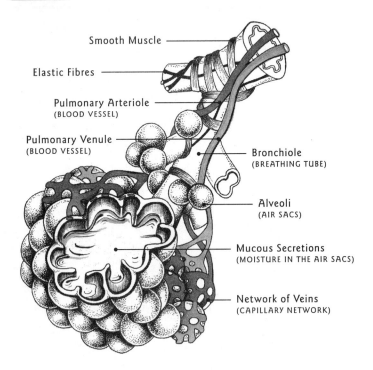

Smooth Muscle

Elastic Fibres

Pulmonary Arteriole
(BLOOD VESSEL)

Pulmonary Venule
(BLOOD VESSEL)

Bronchiole
(BREATHING TUBE)

Alveoli
(AIR SACS)

Mucous Secretions
(MOISTURE IN THE AIR SACS)

Network of Veins
(CAPILLARY NETWORK)

A simplified drawing of part of a healthy lung, which shows how air travels to the air sacs (alveoli). This is a magnified view: the area shown would measure 7 mm. Note especially how the smooth muscle is wrapped around the airways.

DIAGRAM C

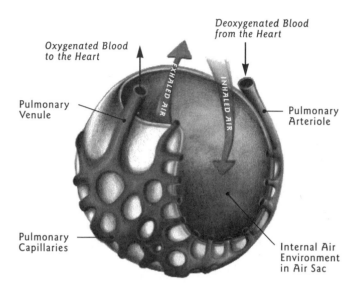

This diagram shows the internal air environment inside one air sac. The shaded arrow on the right shows inhaled air coming in, bringing oxygen and carbon dioxide to mix with the water vapour inside. The air sac retains some oxygen and carbon dioxide for the body's needs, and the rest is breathed out again. Outside the air sac, you can see how the pulmonary arterioles bring blood from the heart to the air sacs. From the air held in each sac, oxygen and carbon dioxide pass into the blood that is flowing through the capillaries (fine blood vessels). From there the blood is taken back to the heart via the pulmonary venules so it can be pumped around the body to feed the tissues.

DIAGRAM D

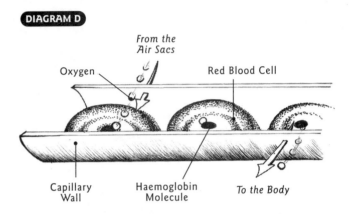

This is a schematic diagram of what happens when oxygen molecules pass from an air sac in the lungs, through the wall of a capillary, and into the blood. The oxygen molecules are absorbed into the red blood cells (left), and when the carbon dioxide level is high enough in the blood, they are better released from the red-cell haemoglobin, through the capillary wall and into the tissues of the body (right). If the carbon dioxide level is not high enough, the oxygen molecule 'sticks' to the haemoglobin molecule (centre) and is trapped in the red cell, and less oxygen is released to feed the tissues.

(continued from page 89)

body tissues. Oxygen is carried in the blood by means of a haemoglobin (Hb) molecule (which is part of a red cell). When carbon dioxide is low due to over-breathing, the oxygen is held tighter than normal to the Hb molecule, due to a chemical bond, and cannot readily come off from the blood. Not enough oxygen is getting into the tissues, so they become starved of oxygen. This oxygen starvation of the tissues is called hypoxia.

The tissues of the human body include muscles. There are three types of muscle:

1. striated muscle e.g. the biceps and triceps muscles
2. smooth muscle: this is found around bronchi and bronchioles or air tubes, around blood vessels, arteries and veins, and as part of the wall of the intestines. You can guess that smooth muscle is of importance in asthma.
3. cardiac muscle (specialised muscle cells, each cell able to contract by itself).

Tissues starved of oxygen cannot be healthy: they become irritable, and the way smooth muscle reacts in distress is to contract, or spasm.

Thus, we start to understand that if carbon dioxide is not at its proper or normal level in the air sacs (6.5%) and falls too low through over-breathing, the oxygen becomes more bound to the haemoglobin molecule and is less able to separate and feed the tissues.

Now, children in the Western world are generally taught that the deeper they breathe, the more oxygen they get 'inside'. Most adults believe this, and in the efficacy of all sorts of 'deep breathing' exercises. It is true that we take in more oxygen when we breathe deeply, but how much oxygen is then available from the blood to the tissues? This availability is governed by something known as the BOHR effect.

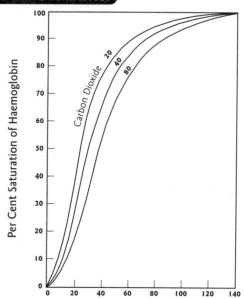

THE VERIGO BOHR EFFECT

Po₂ Partial Pressure (amount) of Oxygen

Haemoglobin-oxygen release (dissociation) is dependent on levels of carbon dioxide. The graph shows what happens in the blood under normal conditions (at 38 °C), at various percentages of oxygen saturation of haemoglobin (represented on the vertical scale). Across the bottom of the graph, levels of oxygen pressure are given. The flowing curves on the graph show different levels of carbon dioxide in the blood (represented as figures of 20, 40 and 80).

To read the graph, take a ruler, place it at any level of Po₂ (oxygen pressure) and draw a line up to the curve showing the lowest level (20) of carbon dioxide. From that point, draw a line straight across to the vertical scale and note the oxygen saturation of haemoglobin. Then note where the original line touches *the highest* CO_2 *(80) and read off the amount on the vertical scale on the left. You will see at once that the* **higher the carbon dioxide** *level, the lower the level of oxygen saturation of haemoglobin — that means* **more oxygen is released to the tissues**. *The* **lower the carbon dioxide** *the tighter the oxygen 'sticks to' the haemoglobin molecule, and the* **less oxygen is released into the tissues**.

The VERIGO-BOHR EFFECT: lowered levels of CO_2 strengthen the bond between haemoglobin and oxygen, thus lowering the oxygenation of the tissues. The stated purpose of the Buteyko method is to reverse the BOHR effect.

To summarise: oxygen enters the lungs, goes into the blood and is trapped by the haemoglobin molecule. How easily it is released, to feed the body cells, depends on the level of carbon dioxide. The oxygen is properly released when carbon dioxide is high in the lungs. If it is low, the tissues suffer oxygen starvation. Oxygen starvation affects all the vital organs, and it has a particular effect in one of them, the brain: it excites the breathing centre located there, setting off a state of breathing stimulation. This increases the breathing even further, creating a 'shortness of breath' sensation in the already over-breathing person, which further deepens the breath. So then there is a further progressive decrease (breathing off) of carbon dioxide from the lungs.

The way to reverse this process is to breathe more shallowly, to trap more carbon dioxide in the lungs and return its level to normal. If the carbon dioxide rises again to normal levels, oxygen is more readily released from the haemoglobin molecules, and can then nourish the tissues and cells.

It is interesting to note that few medical experts in the Western world have taken very much account of the idea of shallow breathing. Eastern ideologies, on the other hand, have proposed for centuries that there is value in stopping over-breathing, and have made breath control part of a wide range of exercises for the body and mind: examples are the practice of meditation, yoga (pranayama breathing), Tai Chi, Chi Gong, and Judd-Shi from Tibet.

Over-breathing, then, is an increase in the function of the lungs above what is normal. It is also called hyperventilation. The significance of Buteyko's discoveries hinges on the diagnosis of what he termed **'hidden hyperventilation'**. This is long-term over-breathing that we are basically not aware of.

Professor Buteyko could clearly see, as can anyone else, the effects of over-breathing to a level of 30 litres of air per minute. Anyone who breathes like this (don't try it!) will suffer the equivalent effect of an acute and serious anxiety attack, i.e. shaking hands, anxiety, chest pain, air hunger, finger tingles and spasm (tetany), cramps, and a racing pulse.

Professor Buteyko became interested in breathing levels in general. What happens, he asked, at all the levels between the extreme hyperventilation we have described, and the normal human breathing rate?

As a reminder, on the opposite page is a repeat of the table on breathing levels from the first chapter of this book.

BREATHING LEVELS

Normal breathing	3 to 5 litres per minute	Healthy level of 6.5% carbon dioxide in air sacs
Hidden over-breathing	5 to 10 litres per minute	Results in very gradual sickness not easily noticed, and illness develops over many years
Over-breathing	10 to 20 litres per minute	This is known as an 'attack', where the adult asthma sufferer, or a person with a related condition, hyperventilates rapidly
Severe over-breathing	20 to 30 litres per minute	At this maximum level, the person suffers a sudden anxiety attack

> *To summarise, over-breathing leads to a lack of carbon dioxide. This lack of carbon dioxide causes an alkaline reaction in the lungs (called respiratory alkalosis).*
> *The body then tries to buffer or balance this situation partially, which sets up a course of events which change the rate and efficiency of activity of all enzyme and vitamin systems (reactions that run our energy and vitality).*

Results of Over-breathing

The ill system that results from the sequence of events shown in the table is obviously going to be more prone to viral illness and allergies, because the shift in the rate of body activity has disturbed the normal flow of chemical reactions in the body and weakened the system.

Looking at these effects, especially the particular effects on the smooth muscles of the body, it is easy to see how over-breathing might cause the following:

- bronchospasm
- spasm of the walls of the arteries
- increased blood pressure

These are identified as symptoms and signs of specific diseases:

- asthma
- angina
- hypertension

You can see how these in turn, if breathing is not corrected, might lead to further *deterioration of asthma, myocardial infarction* (heart attack) and *strokes*.

To understand more about Professor Buteyko's diagnostic theories, turn to the chapter on his life and work. Here, it is sufficient to note that he claims over-breathing to be directly linked to at least 150 diseases.

The diseases that Professor Buteyko has identified as being linked with over-breathing include those overleaf.

- asthma
- emphysema
- allergic rhinitis
- sleep apnoea
- hypertension
- angina
- anxiety
- eczema

The Buteyko theory states that these diseases are the body's defence mechanism against the excessive loss of carbon dioxide through over-breathing.

Defence Mechanisms

To try and guard against this loss of carbon dioxide from the lungs, the human organism has adopted some defence mechanisms:

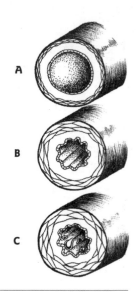

DIAGRAM E

In this diagram, **B** and **C** show what happens inside the airways of an asthma sufferer when the body tissues are starved of oxygen, through lack of carbon dioxide due to over-breathing.

A: The airways are normal and clear, allowing air to move in and out of the passages.

B: The body is reacting to a lack of oxygen in the tissues. The smooth muscles around the airways spasm (tighten) to try to trap carbon dioxide inside the lungs. This is the beginning of an asthma attack.

C: The lining of the airways swells, and mucus clogs up the airways further: the asthma is worsening.

1. Spasm of bronchi and bronchioles. If the airways are in spasm the carbon dioxide cannot easily get out of the body. Thus by narrowing the airways the body can at least maintain a higher level of carbon dioxide, even if it is not the desired 6.5%.

2. Increased mucus and phlegm production. This blocks up the airways to a greater or lesser degree, to keep carbon dioxide concentration at 6.5%, or as high as possible.

3. Swelling of the bronchial wall due to inflammation, further blocking up the airways.

Finally comes the question: what causes the kind of hyperventilation (over-breathing) that leads to serious lowering of carbon dioxide, followed by all these ill effects? Some people seem to over-breathe more than others, so they may be more susceptible to certain external factors. We cannot help them to stop over-breathing until we look at their lifestyle and the factors that exist in their environment, and identify the triggers that may affect them.

The Triggers That Appear to Cause Hyperventilation

According to Professor Buteyko's research, the majority of the population hyperventilates. There are a number of triggers which seem to make this situation a special problem for those who have a tendency towards asthma. They are listed below.

1) The belief that deep breathing is helpful and improves health.

2) Stress, from either positive or negative emotions. Both excitement and depression cause stress. Research carried out by Professor Buteyko shows that people under stress over-breathe.

3) Overeating. One should eat plant protein rather than

animal protein (plant food causes less hyperventilation); raw food more than cooked food (raw food causes less hyperventilation); animal protein, for example red meat and cheese, sharply increases the amount of breathing.

4) Lack of exercise. Lack of physical work or activity leads to overbreathing. Athletes have a low pulse rate (45 to 50), and an athlete or a very fit person will have a slower and shallower breathing rate than the average person. Physical activity encourages the release of carbon dioxide from the cells, increasing its levels in the lungs. The long-term result of fitness is a higher level of carbon dioxide and better nourishment of the body cells.

5) Prolonged sleep. Professor Buteyko has demonstrated that remaining for a long time in a horizontal position, especially lying on the back, causes severe hyperventilation. It is interesting to note that most attacks of epilepsy, asthma, myocardial infarction and strokes occur towards the end of sleep, around 5–6 am. Patients are advised to sleep on the left side, as Professor Buteyko's findings show this causes the least hyperventilation.

6) Heat and stuffy environments (whereas fresh air and cold temperatures assist shallow breathing). This conclusion was reached after over 40 years of measurements.

7) Bronchodilators. These give quick initial relief to someone having an asthma attack, as they are designed to

open the airways. By increasing the patient's capacity to over-breathe, however, in effect they can perpetuate hyperventilation, which, as the Professor argues, further aggravates asthma.

8) Smoking, excessive alcohol and other stress-provoking factors, including excessive sexual activity.

In this book we are concentrating on the effective treatment of asthma, since it is so prevalent in our society and the results of the method have been so spectacularly successful over so many years. But from reading this chapter and the case histories in the previous chapter, it is easy to see that the method may be of use against a wide variety of diseases. The simple aim of the Buteyko method is to reduce the patient's total volume of air breathed to normal levels per minute. The normal average volume of air breathed by an adult is 3 to 4 litres per minute.

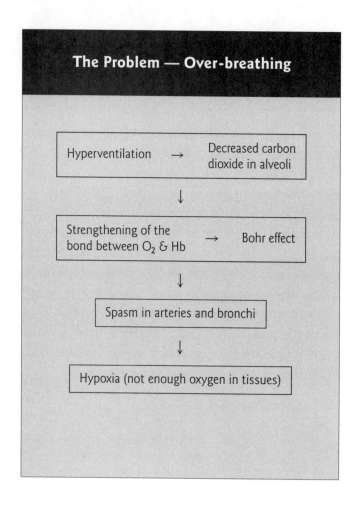

The Problem — Over-breathing

Hyperventilation → Decreased carbon dioxide in alveoli

↓

Strengthening of the bond between O_2 & Hb → Bohr effect

↓

Spasm in arteries and bronchi

↓

Hypoxia (not enough oxygen in tissues)

The Solution — Breathing Less, and More Shallowly

Hypoventilation (shallower breathing) $\rightarrow$ CO_2 increases in air sacs

$\downarrow$

Weakening of bond between O_2 and Hb (Hb less 'sticky')

$\downarrow$

Better oxygenation of tissues

$\downarrow$

- Blood pressure decreases
- Asthma decreases
- Angina decreases

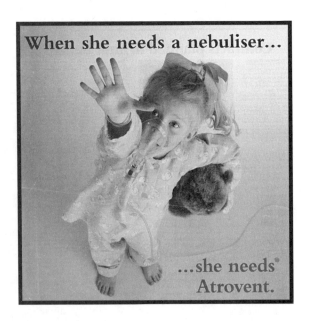

Treatment of Asthma with Drugs

Current Approaches

This book would not be complete without a description of the drugs that are currently prescribed for the treatment of asthma. Most asthmatics take particular medication over a period of time, and change this medication occasionally on the advice of their medical practitioner. Doctors select medication from the range available at the time, taking all factors into account, and deciding on what they consider is best for their patient. For a number of reasons, including the complexity of the actual drugs prescribed, asthma sufferers (or the parents of children who suffer from asthma) do not always have a clear idea about a particular drug, how it works, or what its recognised side effects may be. This chapter is devoted to the current range of drugs so that asthma sufferers can take a closer look at the nature of the medication they may be taking, and the purposes for which it is prescribed.

Drugs for the treatment of asthma are commonly known as maintenance drugs. This is because they do not cure asthma: they are intended to keep it at bay. Such drugs have traditionally been considered the best possible medical and scientific approach to helping sufferers control their asthma, especially for moderate and severe asthma, for which frequent or regular therapy is necessary.

It is important to understand the nature of these drugs and the way they operate in the body over the long term, especially since few asthma sufferers these days are prescribed only one drug — most use two types: bronchodilators and anti-inflammatory drugs.

TABLE I

SUMMARY OF DRUGS USED IN ASTHMA		
Drug	**Mode of Action**	**Administration**
Sodium cromo-glycate	Anti-inflammatory	Inhaled
Corticosteroids	Anti-inflammatory	Inhaled/oral
Beta-Agonists *short-acting* *long-acting*	Bronchodilator	Injected Inhaled/oral Inhaled/oral
Anti-cholinergics	Bronchodilator	Inhaled
Xanthines	Bronchodilator, *weak anti-inflammatory*	Oral/rectal/ injected

TABLE 2

BRONCHODILATORS	
Drug	**Brand Name**
Bronchodilators	
Beta Agonists:	
Fenoterol	Berotec MDI
Orciprenaline	Alupent MDI
Salbutamol	Asmol MDI
	Respolin MDI
	Ventolin MDI
	Ventolin Rotocaps
	Ventolin tabs
	Ventolin syrup
Salmeterol	Serevent MDI
Serevent disks	
Terbutaline	Bricanyl MDI
	Bricanyl Turbuhaler
	Bricanyl tabs
	Bricanyl elixir
Anticholinergics	
Ipratropium bromide	Atrovent MDI

Bronchodilators or Relievers

These are the Beta-agonist and anticholinergic bronchodilators listed in Table 2 above. They are useful in relieving attacks, since they are designed to open the airways and keep them open for a period of hours, giving a feeling of relief.

■ MEDICINE

Asthma: The Hidden Killer

Model Krissy Taylor's death underscores how lethal and deceptive this common ailment can be

By CHRISTINE GORMAN

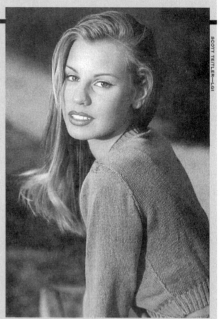

A LIFE CUT SHORT: An autopsy finally detects the ailment the 17-year-old beauty didn't know she had

AT FIRST THE CORONER COULD NOT tell what killed Krissy Taylor, the 17-year-old model who died mysteriously in her Florida home four weeks ago. Krissy's lungs appeared to be normal. Her heart seemed fine. There was no sign of alcohol, cocaine, amphetamines or other drugs in her blood. But when the pathologist looked through a microscope at tissue samples from the teenager's body, he noted that the bronchioles, the tiniest airways in the lungs, were inflamed and scarred. These telltale signs, he reported last week, indicated that Taylor, like more than 6,000 other Americans each year, had died of a fairly common ailment: asthma.

In addition, Taylor treated her symptoms with an over-the-counter remedy—in this case, Primatene Mist—that probably masked the severity of her condition. Despite warning labels that clearly state no one should use the inhaler unless a doctor has diagnosed asthma, Taylor depended on it to alleviate her occasional shortness of breath. Such self-treatment frustrates doctors. "Every time people use these over-the-counter remedies, they are delaying getting long-term care," says Busse.

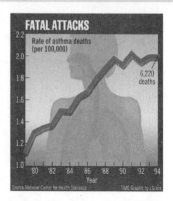

Sections from an article in TIME *magazine, 7 August 1995.*

Side Effects of Beta-agonist Bronchodilators

When these drugs are used, there are a number of side effects which are known to the medical profession and described clearly in the information available to those who dispense the medication. The summaries given here are drawn from that published information. Patients are usually warned about some of these side effects. But there are others that the patient will be less conscious of at first. These accepted side effects are:

- hyperventilation
- tremor in muscles (often felt as a shaking of the hands)
- restlessness
- headache
- palpitations, tachycardia (fast heartbeat)
- gastrointestinal upset (indigestion)
- dizziness
- hypokalaemia (lowering of the potassium level which in turn, can lead to weakness, fatigue and irregular heart rhythm).

Side Effects of Anticholinergic Bronchodilators

These drugs have the following recognised side effects:

- dry mouth
- urinary retention

- acute-angle glaucoma (increased pressure within the eyeball, which can lead to blindness)
- throat irritation
- accommodation disturbances (difficulty in focussing the eyes)

Dangers of Beta-agonist Bronchodilators

Most people who have asthma or have had anything to do with an asthma sufferer will have become aware over the last few years of the fears (in both medical circles and

This puffer's cool

WILL Bart Simpson triumph where so many parents and practitioners have struggled?

The National Asthma Campaign is hoping his unmistakeable mug will help convince young patients to comply with their asthma inhaler medication.

That's why they've endorsed the Puffa Pal (pictured), which will fit over most brands of inhaler and sells at pharmacies for $4.95.

It is their hope that it may reduce part of the stigma associated with inhaler medication used by children.

Youngsters (or perhaps the young at heart) can take their pick from Bart, Lisa and Homer Simpson, with other characters such as Spiderman, Daffy Duck, Tweety, The Tasmanian Devil, and a glow-in-the-dark Casper to be available later this year. MO

Rachel Sharp

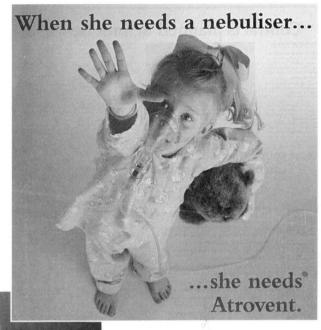

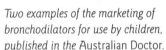

*Two examples of the marketing of
bronchodilators for use by children,
published in the* Australian Doctor.

in the public arena) about the possibly dangerous side effects of Beta-agonist bronchodilators. A number of scientific tests have been made to examine these.

In the late 1980s the Saskatchewan Asthma Epidemiology Project in the USA showed a close-related association between the use of Beta-agonists and death or near death from asthma.

In 1989 a study was published in the British medical journal, the *Lancet* — this was the first major case-controlled study assessing the role of anti-asthmatic drugs in asthma mortality in New Zealand. The study included 12,301 patients. The Cohort covered 47,842 person years of follow-up.

The study concluded that long-term use of Beta-agonist bronchodilators, particularly the protracted use of Fenoterol and Salbutamol, was associated with an increased risk of asthma-related death or near death. The increased risk of fatal and near fatal asthma with these Beta-agonists was clinically important for patients who used more than one or two canisters per month.

For patients who used more than two canisters per month alone (that is, without cortisone treatments), both bronchodilators were associated with a greatly increased risk of death, which was especially marked for Fenoterol.

This information is worrying when one considers that in some countries bronchodilators are obtainable over the counter without a doctor's prescription. Thus asthma patients, particularly mild asthmatics who do not want to have to attend a doctor regularly about their recurring and familiar ailment, are virtually treating themselves for their condition. In these circumstances their use of bronchodilators is unlikely to be adequately observed or controlled, because there may be no one to inform them that they should use anti-inflammatory agents, or preventers.

In the USA, almost one million Americans between the ages of 13 and 34 suffer from asthma. Sales of bronchodilators are high for this age group, and marketing is keen — to the extent that new puffers are being aimed specifically at teenagers. Designers have added graffiti to inhalers and come up with a hot-rod and a dragon inhaler, to mention just two. The performer Aphex Twin once used an inhaler as a pop-culture icon in his video dance-hall hit, 'Ventolin'. In other markets such as Australia, the images of popular television figures and toys are used to encourage younger children to accept medication by bronchodilators.

From our understanding of the Buteyko theory about the underlying cause of asthma, we can see why bronchodilators might be dangerous, if by opening the airways they encourage the asthma sufferer to over-breathe. In previous chapters, we have seen that the body uses defence mechanisms against the loss of CO_2 from the lungs caused by over-breathing, and these defence mechanisms start to be used when CO_2 levels reach between 5–5.5% or below, in the alveoli (tiny air sacs in the lungs). The defence mechanisms to stop the effects of hyperventilation include those listed overleaf.

1.Spasm of the airways to keep the CO_2 in the lung and prevent it from being breathed off to the atmosphere by over-breathing,

2.Mucus production to further protect the lungs from CO_2 loss (further blockage),

3.Inflammation within the bronchial walls causing further constriction to reduce CO_2 loss.

Unfortunately, these defence mechanisms make the person more wheezy and sick, and may indicate that the asthma is worsening. It is thus possible to see how, according to Buteyko theory, the use of bronchodilators may contribute to a deterioration in an asthma sufferer's condition.

In recent years the death rate from asthma worldwide has escalated alarmingly. In Australia, for instance, there was a high of 900 deaths annually in the late 1980s. In the 1990s, the death rate is around 800 per year. The increase in deaths from asthma throughout Western countries since 1980s has caused some commentators to speak of an 'epidemic' of asthma. An article in Britain's *New Scientist* of 6 April 1991 carried the headline: ARE ASTHMA DRUGS THE CURE THAT KILLS? It said:

There is no doubt that beta-2 agonists, usually inhaled as a fine spray or powder, are the best short-term treatment for an asthma attack. Their effect is felt in a couple of minutes, bringing welcome relief from even severe attacks. But some doctors now wonder if asthmatics are paying a price for this immediate relief. Between 1980 and 1988, deaths from asthma in Britain rose from 1500 a year up to 2000 a year... Similar increases have been charted in New Zealand, Germany and Scandinavian countries. Meanwhile, the number of prescriptions for beta-2 agonists has risen from 8 million a year to 15 million a year in Britain. The question is whether the drugs are contributing to the rise in the death rate.

Partly because of such concerns, it has become medical practice worldwide to establish a rule that anyone who uses a bronchodilator often or regularly must use a 'preventative' drug, generally cortisone spray or cortisone tablets. These drugs are called 'preventative' because they are intended to reduce the extra inflammation caused by the bronchodilators.

Despite these cautionary measures, more bronchodilators continued to be released. In the 1990s, for instance, long-acting (up to 12 hours) bronchodilators such as Serevent (Salmeterol Xinafoate) were released in Australia.

What are the 'Preventatives'?

Steroids

Steroids, or glucocorticoids, are potent anti-inflammatory agents which decrease the number of white cells, inhibit activated T lymphocytes and suppress many other aspects of the inflammatory response. They do suppress inflammation but reduce the body's ability to fight infection.

Steroids have a number of side effects, recognised by the medical profession. The acute side effects are:

- weight gain and appetite stimulation
- nervousness, irritability up to mania, ADD-like syndrome in children (ADD is Attention Deficit Disorder)

THE EARLY use of low-dose inhaled corticosteroids in patients with mild to moderate asthma was widely supported at a recent meeting of Australian and New Zealand respiratory specialists in Melbourne. "There's no doubt that steroids are the most effective therapy for asthma currently available, and should be considered as first line treatment for patients with chronic asthma," said **Professor Peter Barnes**, from the National Heart and Lung Institute in London.

Professor Paul O'Byrne, Professor of Respiratory Medicine at McMaster University in Canada, reported on a general practice study of patients with asthma which their doctors considered was 'too mild' to warrant the use of inhaled corticosteroids. However, when they were started on treatment the benefits were substantial.

Prof Peter Barnes

Part of an article from Australian Doctor, 16 April 1993, which reflects acceptance of the use of cortisone, even in mild asthma.

- hyperglycaemia (blood sugar goes higher than normal, but is reversible), diabetes
- salt and water retention
- gastric irritation
- blurred vision
- hoarseness and/or throat irritation.

TABLE 3

PREVENTATIVES	
Anti-inflammatories	**Brand Name**
Corticosteroids	
Oral	
Prednisolone	Various brands
Prednisone	
Cortisone acetate	
Inhaled	
Beclomethasone	Aldecin MDI
Diproprionate	Becotide MDI
	Becloforte MDI
	Becotide Rotacaps
Budesonide	Pulmicort MDI
	Pulmicort Turbuhaler
Sodium cromoglycate	
	Intal MDI
	Intal Forte MDI
	Intal Spincaps
Medocromil	Tilade

The chronic side effects (those produced over time) are:
- cataracts
- osteoporosis (thinning and crumbling of bones)
- myopathy (muscle pain) due to muscle damage
- oral candidiasis (oral thrush) up to 40%
- damage to and thinning of the skin, and tendency to bruising
- depression
- hypothalamic pituitary adrenal axis depression (upset of hormonal balance in the body).
- growth retardation in children — due to an acceleration of epiphyseal closure (ends of body stop growing abnormally early)

One of the more dangerous side effects of steroids has been mentioned — this is the hypothalamic pituitary adrenal axis depression, which means that the natural production of steroid is suppressed. The body knows it is receiving extra steroid artificially from outside and that

Drug trial offers hope

A DRUG to stop asthma attacks is being trialled in Sydney.

If it is effective, the drug will be a major breakthrough in stopping asthma before it develops, a respiratory expert said yesterday.

Director of clinical trials at Sydney's Royal North Shore Hospital, Dr David Allen, said inflammation of the airways was the major cause of asthma.

The new medication blocked the inflammatory reaction rather than suppressing it as current drugs did, he said.

"If tests find this drug is effective, it will

By KATRINA BEIKOFF

mean great things for asthma sufferers, Dr Allen said.

"The asthma will be cut off before it gets a chance to really develop. It's a new angle on what we're already able to do."

The Japanese manufactured drug — a leukotrienne antagonist — will undergo simultaneous trials in Sydney, Europe and South Africa.

It has already been trialled in Japan bu

there are plenty of steroids in the blood — so it shuts down its own production. This is fine in ordinary 'smooth' living, but in an emergency, such as serious infection, surgery or injury, steroids essential in the fear-fright-flight reaction cannot be produced to the degree needed.

Even in inhaled-only steroids, for anyone taking more than 800 mcg per day there is a dose-dependent incidence of oral and throat candidiasis (the author theorises that generalised intestinal candidiasis may also develop).

Dysphonia is a term meaning the inability to form proper vocal sounds. This can happen to people taking steroids, and it is thought to be due to temporary damage to the nerves supplying the larynx (vagus nerves) as well as being due to local irritation. Unilateral (one-sided) vocal cord paralysis has been described in some patients.

for asthma

the effectiveness and correct dosage for Westerners has not yet been set.

Dr Allen said the hospital was looking for asthmatics to help trial the drug.

"The lack of side-effects also gives great hope to asthma sufferers," Dr Allen said.

"Current treatments involve taking steroids to suppress the inflammation.

"Steroids can cause weight gain, high blood pressure, fluid retention and osteoporosis. If these tablets are effective they could be on the market in two years — that's great news for asthmatics."

A news article from The Daily Telegraph Mirror, *28 July 1994, reflecting the continued search for alternatives to steroids in asthma treatment.*

Sodium Cromoglycate (Intal) and Medocromil (Tilade)

These agents play a smaller part as 'preventatives'. They inhibit inflammatory cells in asthma and are considered the least harmful agents used. Their limited side effects are throat and tracheal irritation, rash and cough. Tilade appears to have an increased effectiveness in adults whereas Intal is more effective in children than adults.

Xanthines

These agents are often referred to as 'the other bronchodilators' mainly because they do in fact cause less bronchodilation than those in Table 1, but also because of their potentially severe side-effects which include:

- gastrointestinal upsets: nausea, reflux, diarrhoea
- headache
- dizziness
- palpitation (irregular heartbeat or 'beating of the chest')
- (fast heart and pulse rhythm)
- arrhythmia (dangerous, irregular beating of the heart)
- convulsions (at higher blood levels).

Antibiotics

Antibiotics have little place in asthma prevention and treatment as (generally) bacterial infections cause little

TABLE 4

THE XANTHINES	
Xanthine	**Brand Name**
Theophylline	Austyn caps
	Elixophyllin elixir
	Nuelin tabs
	Nuelin syrup
	Nuelin SR
	Nuelin Sprinkle
	Sio-Bid caps
	Theo-Dur tabs
Aminophylline	Cardophyllin suppositories
Choline	Brondecon expectorant
theophyllinate	and elixir
	Brondecon PD tabs
	Choledyl tabs

wheeze and most 'wheezy' attacks are caused by viruses, allergy or emotional stress. Antibiotics do play a part, though, in chronic bronchitis, emphysema and sinusitis. Antibiotics kill bacteria but have no effect on viruses. The common side effects of antibiotics are:

- oral candida (thrush)
- vaginal candida infection
- bowel candida infection (not generally accepted)
- allergic responses such as (skin) rashes
- life-threatening reactions such as liver failure and anaphylaxis, which is choking and swelling of the throat and body.

Mucolytics
Mucolytics are agents which thin mucus. These are used to decrease the blockage of the airways that mucus causes, and relieve the asthma patient's discomfort.

Antihistamines
Antihistamines have no real value in asthma treatment as they dry secretions and cause dry mucus plugging of airways.

Does the Asthma Sufferer Have an Alternative to Drugs?

The Buteyko method offers the only effective alternative that I have seen, to continued treatment of asthma by drugs alone. Buteyko practitioners have observed that most people can control their asthma by undergoing a course of simple Buteyko exercises over five to seven sessions (even a child over four-and-a-half is easily able to undergo the course). As we have mentioned, the exercises have also been shown to benefit those suffering from other respiratory conditions such as allergic rhinitis, emphysema, chronic bronchitis and sleep apnoea.

What Happens to Drug Treatment When You Undertake the Method?

During the classes at the clinic, practitioners insist that a patient, under supervision, must reduce the use of bronchodilators as soon as possible, because according to the Professor's theory they cause the asthma to worsen by causing hyperventilation. Steroids, however, are often retained at first to control the symptoms, and they may even be increased briefly and temporarily, to enable the patient to achieve the best pauses from his/her lessons.

As soon as progress is made, the inhaled or oral steroids are gradually and responsibly withdrawn under a practitioner's and a doctor's supervision.

Most patients using the Buteyko technique find that their symptoms begin to disappear so that they need fewer and fewer drugs, and finally none at all. These people are gaining relief from asthma and also from the side effects of the drugs that we have described above. The benefits are wonderful. Many moderate to severe asthmatics, after practising the Buteyko exercises as regularly as they are advised to do, testify to their rapid weight loss and loss of irritability. They find that they are more relaxed and their mood improves greatly. Many parents of children who have learned to control their asthma in this way, say that their children are happier, more manageable and more responsive, and that their school results escalate.

Some patients who have had severe asthma, however, even after they have achieved significant control and thus cut down their drug intake, are unfortunately left with some bone osteoporosis due to their steroid intake (the author has seen this even in teenagers, in whom it is difficult to remedy).

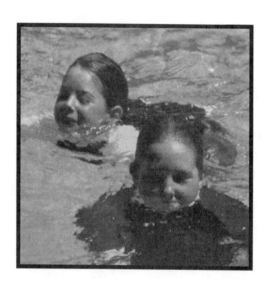

Asthma and Naturopathy

Other Treatments for Asthma

The Buteyko method stands alone as an effective long-term treatment for asthma, but it should be further enhanced by basic naturopathic health rules. Because poor diet, stress and the chemicals in medications and the environment are the main external triggers in the onset of ill health, their correction is vital to a full recovery. The ways to correct them, in order of importance are:

1. Strict adherence to diet and the reduction of allergy-provoking agents
2. A reduction in the level of stress, plus adequate rest and relaxation
3. Appropriately prescribed nutritional supplements — oral or injected
4. Adequate gentle exercise
5. Other helpful therapies.

OPPOSITE PAGE: *Both traditional medical advice and Buteyko recommend swimming as the best exercise for asthmatics.*

Diet

First and foremost, remember that overeating causes over-breathing. Secondly, remember that one-third of what we eat feeds us; the other two-thirds feeds the doctor.

There are a number of dietary considerations specific to asthma and other respiratory conditions. Professor Buteyko has calculated, after years of measurements, that eating *meat* produces more hyperventilation than eating vegetables. *Cooked food* produces more hyperventilation than raw food.

If specific allergies have been diagnosed in your case, of course you will take account of these also in planning your diet (see the allergy section below).

Over-eating leads to hyperventilation, which leads to asthma. A vegetarian diet is best for asthmatics. If you suffer from asthma, the following guidelines will help you. Avoid all meat and fish as an initial step when replanning your diet. Avoid cow's milk. Goat's milk is well tolerated, especially in soured form as yoghurt. So is soy milk. You should try to eat lots of garlic and green vegetables and all available fruits plus natural, unfiltered honey. Pollen when inhaled is an irritant, but taken orally by capsule or as an ingredient of honey, it actually prevents allergy. Eat plenty of raw seeds and nuts, and sprouted seeds and grains. Wheat products are best avoided initially, as many individuals who suffer from asthma are allergic to them. The diet should include manganese-rich foods such as peas, beans, blueberries, nuts, buckwheat. It is believed that chronic manganese deficiency may be one of the contributing causes of asthma.

Asthma sufferers are advised to spice up their meals. Small amounts of chillies, cayenne, ginger, curry and garlic in the diet make coughing easier and mucus thinner. Recently, omega 3 fish oils have been found to alleviate asthma.

It is beneficial to take lemon juice in a teaspoon of water three times daily. It helps to break up mucus and is rich in vitamin C.

The Low-Stress Diet

This diet is helpful, but not specific, for people who suffer from asthma. Basically, it entails the strict avoidance of the following:

1. Sugar-rich foods, e.g.: confectionery, soft drinks, glucose, malt, foods containing cane sugar such as sweet biscuits, cakes, desserts, golden syrup, molasses, dried fruits, sweet dried fruits. Fruit juices should be diluted 50% with mineral water or preferably purified water, and you should not drink more than two glasses of diluted juice per day. By avoiding all of the above you will be helping your body correct hypoglycaemia (low blood sugar). This is important, especially as a way to alleviate nocturnal asthma.

2. White flour products and refined starchy foods such as white bread, biscuits, non-wholemeal pasta, pastries, pies, sauces, gravies and canned and bottled foods which may contain white flour as a filling or bulking agent.

Asthma less likely in children who eat fish

A DIET rich in oily fish such as salmon may dramatically reduce the risk of a child developing asthma, according to the results of a survey of children aged 8-11.

Linda Hodge, a dietitian at the Institute of Respiratory Medicine at Sydney's Royal Prince Alfred Hospital, presented the findings to a meeting of the Thoracic Society of Australia and New Zealand in Hobart.

The survey showed that children with a high consumption of oily fish had one-fifth the risk of developing asthma compared with those with a diet low in these foods.

Ms Hodge said the results supported a protective role of fish which first emerged from a study of asthma risk factors in 1993. However, the earlier study could not determine whether fish intake was a marker for some other aspect of the diet — such as sodium, selenium, magnesium or antioxidant vitamins — which might play a role in asthma.

The latest findings were based on dietary questionnaires returned by the parents of 484 children who had been assessed for airway hyper-responsiveness, atopy and recent wheeze. About 58% had normal airways, 16% had wheeze, 11% had airway hyper-responsiveness and 15% had asthma, defined as the presence of both wheeze and airway hyper-responsiveness.

There was no difference between asthmatics and non-asthmatics in intake of any of the nutrients assessed, including selenium, sodium, magnesium and the antioxidant vitamins, nor in any of

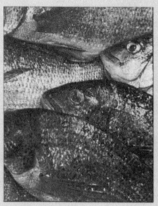

the 200 foods analysed, except for the intake of fresh fish.

Children with asthma ate only about 7g per week of oily fish, compared with 30g per week in controls. After adjusting for factors such as atopy, parental history of asthma or smoking, and respiratory infections in the first two years of life, children with a higher consumption of oily fish had only one-fifth the risk of developing asthma.

Ms Hodge said the eicosanoids, produced by the metabolism of omega-3 fatty acids in fish oil, were less inflammatory and less likely to cause smooth muscle spasm than their counterparts produced from omega-6 fatty acids, which were found in high concentrations in oils used to manufacture margarine. Whether by-products from omega-3 fatty acids had an anti-inflammatory effect was still being investigated.

— Tony James

3. Coffee and conventional tea. These are unnecessary stimulants which have been shown to increase levels of anxiety, thus interfering with any attempts to reduce stress in the unwell person. Coffee has also been proven to raise cholesterol levels in the blood. Preferably, drink three to six glasses per day of 'purified', filtered tap water and herbal teas. Remember that mucus tends to be thicker when you are dehydrated.

4. All alcoholic beverages, as alcohol is toxic, and therefore a stress factor. Many people are allergic to wine additives, though red wine is rich in antioxidant vitamins, due to the inclusion of grape skins and seeds.

5. All tobacco products, all cigarette smoke (including 'passive' smoke), all drugs (unless medically prescribed). Try to avoid environmental pollutants, including chemicals at work and in the home. Inspect food packaging to avoid harmful additives.

6. Try to cut down on cooked food in your diet. Eat fresh, organically grown fruits and vegetables: at least one third of the vegetables should be eaten raw. When you do cook food, lightly steam or stir-fry it. Avoid hidden sugars in desserts, and in processed foods such as canned fruits, baked beans, breakfast cereals.

OPPOSITE PAGE: *An article that appeared in Australian Doctor on 14 April 1995.*

Alternative Choices For Diet-conscious Asthmatics

1. Tap water	*Purified tap water or low salt mineral water, three to six glasses daily*
2. Tea and Coffee	*Herbal teas and dandelion coffee*
3. Sugar	*Fruits and diluted fruit juices*
4. Chocolate	*Carob powder in small quantities*
5. Smoking and Alcohol	*Replace with positive, health-giving habits and activities. (Use acupuncture to stop these habits.)*

Allergies

Many people have sensitivities to foods and chemicals which manifest themselves in a wide range of symptoms, including those of asthma. Needless to say, such foods should be avoided. Allergy testing may need to be performed to discover all of a patient's allergies.

Orthodox allergy specialists carry out blood RAST and/or skin prick tests. These generally give limited results, but they may reveal that the individual is sensitive to things such as: pollens, dust, dust mites, animal danders and a limited food profile — milk, eggs, citrus, wheat etc. On the RAST test these are graded as 0–5. 0–1 results are negative or equivocal, 2–5 are considered to be significant.

Skin Prick Test

In a skin prick test, the size of the skin reaction (or weal) produced on the skin indicates the amount of allergy. Specialists can then make up dilutions of the allergy-provoking substance of differing strengths, and administer these in slightly increasing amounts orally, or by injection under the skin. This is called desensitisation. It is time-consuming (it can take months or years) and relatively costly, but effective in some individuals.

Recently, alternative allergy tests have become popular, and it is important to know what they involve. Three of them are listed on the following pages, with details about how they provide information.

Dr Coca Test

This simplest of all tests measures one's increase in pulse rate after eating a certain allergenic food or being exposed to a certain chemical allergen. To obtain a measurement, the rise or fall in an individual's pulse rate is recorded, up to 90 minutes after eating certain foods. A normal pulse rate is about 70 per minute. The rate may rise to 160 per minute in such a test, which indicates a severe case of allergy.

It should be added that the Buteyko method often alleviates allergy.

It is the author's experience that many allergies, present before the course of breathing exercises, vanish as people familiarise themselves with the exercises and stop their hyperventilation. As we noted, in addition to the pulse rate rising the level and rate of breathing also rapidly rises when the person is challenged with a reactive food.

Vega Test (also called Mora test, Thera test, Electrodermal testing, Listen machine)

This method comes from Germany and tests allergies according to acupuncture meridians. The test is experimental at this stage, but over the last 10 years, more alternative practitioners are using this form of allergy testing to obtain additional information. Two or more pages of information are gathered after the test, including food and chemical allergies graded from 0–100. The lower the score, the stronger the allergy.

This test also provides information about the likelihood of candida and its severity, as well as measuring the condition of vital organs. Vitamin and mineral deficiencies are clearly shown after this test, and the levels of heavy metals in the body are depicted. The test takes thirty minutes and costs are usually under $50. A more extensive version of this test takes one hour and costs under $100 (Australian figures in 1997).

The Bryan's Cytotoxic Test

This test is carried out in Australia by the Australian Biologic's testing services. This examines some 70 foods, food additives, fungi and antibiotics, and shows the range of allergy to these. This test costs about $80 (Australian figures, 1997).

Vitamins and Minerals

Your doctor may advise some of the following to build up your lungs and immune system:

- Vitamin C. This is the main anti-oxidant, immune enhancer, anti-inflammatory agent. There are some 72,000 chemicals which can damage our body cells by oxidation, which is rather like the process of rusting or going rancid within our body — anti-oxidants like vitamin C help to prevent this. It promotes healing of lung tissue, protects against chemicals, detoxifies the cells, helps prevent infection. Thirteen out of 19 papers reviewed by the Australian College of Nutritional and Environmental Medicine (of which the author is a Fellow) show benefit/remission of asthma after supplementing with Vitamin C.
- Bioflavonoids. These are a part of the Vitamin C com-

plex. They alter membrane permeability (lower the rate at which the bronchial wall swells), and stimulate lymphocytes to produce interferon (a virus fighter). Quercetin (one of the bioflavonoids) has been shown to be a MAST cell inhibitor (that is, it inhibits one of the cells shown to cause inflammation in asthma).

- Vitamins A and D. These are specific for mucus membranes. The recommended doses per day to normalise the function of the mucus membranes are: vitamin A 21,000 Iu (International units), Vitamin D 1000 Iu. (Doses of Vitamin A above 2500 Iu per day should be avoided in pregnancy.)
- Vitamin E. This oxygenates the blood and acts as an antioxidant. The recommended dose is 500–750 Iu daily.
- Zinc. This is an immune enhancer and anti-oxidant. A beneficial daily dose is 30 mg.
- Magnesium. This is a bronchial muscle antispasmodic (relaxes airways). The dose is 45 mg daily.
- Selenium. This is an anti-oxidant. The dose is 400 mcg per day.
- B complex vitamins. These are necessary to build up the nervous system and alleviate stress, specifically oral B6, which should be taken in doses of 50–100 mg daily, and B12, which should be taken orally or by injection in 100–5000 mcg doses twice weekly. High doses of B12 vitamins, injected daily, have been shown in clinical trials to alleviate asthma in children in the USA, though the doctor conducting the therapy noted that the benefits ceased when the injections were stopped.

Vitamin Injection

A special program of vitamin injections is available to enable most patients to feel the benefits of nutritional therapies. When some of the supplements are administered by injection, problems of poor absorption are overcome. Also, there is no stomach or bowel irritation. The injections generally produce minimal pain and are well tolerated by most patients, as they regard the discomfort as insignificant when compared to the often rapid improvement in well-being they provide. Injection therapy, if prescribed, is of the utmost importance in recovery from illness, and maintenance of optimal good health.

Vitamin C is injected intravenously (12.5 g to 30 g in a straight push, and 30 g to 90 g by intravenous drip), and Vitamin B complex with B12 (1000 mcg) is injected intramuscularly, once or twice a week for a course of injections. Magnesium sulphate ($Mg\ SO_4$) can be injected intramuscularly to alleviate spasm. One 5 ml ampoule containing a dose of 2.47 g is given once to three times weekly.

Stress Reduction and Rest

These are vitally important for a full and lasting recovery from any illness. Recurrent stress may cause a return of symptoms. Try to identify the problem areas. Steps should be taken to reduce overwork and resolve conflicts. Yoga, relaxation, counselling, personal growth psychotherapy and meditation may be helpful. A quarter of asthma sufferers have a deep-seated nervous or emotional problem. Stress leads to hyperventilation, so it must be reduced by a variety of means. The Buteyko method is particularly useful in relieving anxiety, and can help even people who suffer severe panic attacks.

Exercise

Brisk walking, light jogging, cycling and swimming are ideal exercises and should be undertaken for half an hour daily, preferably after some Buteyko courses. Low-impact aerobics are also excellent. If you have not exercised regu-

Asthmatic kids take to water

AN evaluation of a purpose-designed swimming program for asthmatic children was presented to delegates.

Colleen Wardell, of the Asthma Foundation of New South Wales, said the program was established 30 years ago and anecdotal evidence of its success was formally examined in 1994.

Pre- and post-evaluation surveys were conducted for at least 12 months and included 73 children and 20 instructors.

Significant improvements were recorded in participants' quality of life; 77% of them reported increased self-confidence, 74% reported a reduced absence from school, 46% reported fewer visits to doctors, and 64% reported fewer visits to hospitals.

Children who took part in the program showed an increased awareness and understanding of their condition. They had also learned how to relax and to enjoy sport and not to feel disadvantaged by their asthma.

While there was no demonstrable change in PEFR attributable to the program, there was an indication of a shift from reliever medications such as bronchodilators to preventive inhaled steroids. PH

larly, start with five minutes and slowly build up to 30 minutes daily. It is a good idea to do five minutes of warm-up exercises before commencing each session. Try to exercise enough to feel 'good' after each session rather than puffed out and tired. Learn to read your body and mind — to perceive the true nature of your physical being, what it likes and dislikes. Be aware that in some people, jogging and cycling may trigger their asthma.

The best sport for asthma is regular swimming. Many respiratory specialists recommend swimming as helpful or curative without realising that they are stopping hyper-ventilation. They are advocating hypoventilation (decreased breathing) under the stress of exercise, which actively

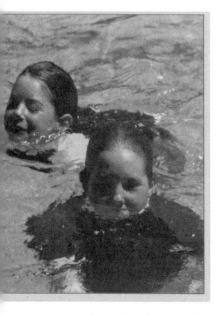

An article from the Medical Observer *of 18 April 1997.*

raises the level of CO_2 gas in the lungs and blood vessels, exactly as the Buteyko exercises do. Such advisers are in fact recommending the Buteyko method without realising it.

The advantage of the Buteyko practice, once you have received the instruction in the method, is that it can be carried out in your own home, in your own time, without expending the energy necessary in swimming. But there are many benefits in regular exercise: an improved feeling of well-being, the stimulation of the production of endorphin (the 'good feeling' hormone in our bodies that also has an anti-inflammatory effect), reduction in anxiety and depression, normalising blood sugar levels and weight, relieving arthritis pain and increasing energy levels.

Herbal Treatment

If your doctor thinks it beneficial, he or she may gradually introduce herbal tablets or liquids to complement, or substitute for your drug treatment. Herbs generally have fewer side effects than most drugs. Herbs often used include grindelia, echinacea, euphorbia, garlic, passiflora, drosera, licorice, thuja, mint and ginkgo biloba.

Homoeopathic Agents

Your naturopath may recommend some of the following: ipecac, arsenicum album, natrum sulph.

Chiropractic/Osteopathic Adjustments

These can relieve pressure on the nerves that control the lungs. Manipulation is directed to relaxing the T3–T4 area in the upper spine just below the neck, from which nerve messages are sent to the lungs. They can also alter habitual neuromuscular patterns associated with hyperventilation. Furthermore, adjustments can correct:

1. elevated ribs (many asthmatics develop an enlarged, expanded chest, while people with emphysema develop a 'barrel' chest)
2. kyphosis (abnormal bend in the spine)
3. neck, shoulder muscle contraction (these are accessory or extra muscles of respiration)
4. muscle spasm around the diaphragm.

Acupuncture

Acupuncture in Eastern medicine has been used for more than 3,000 years to alleviate asthma.

Acupuncture with needles or low-power laser can be a powerful tool in relieving airway spasms, sometimes permanently. The author has many asthma patients who after 1–3 courses of acupuncture (each of 8 –12 treatments) have maintained a state of well-being for years.

Shiatsu

This technique of massage and finger pressure has become popular due to the fact that needles are not necessary. Similar points to those chosen in acupuncture are massaged and stimulated by finger pressure.

Chi Gong and Tai Chi

These are old and proven routines of body and breathing exercises that alleviate asthma. The breathing is slow and rhythmic, designed to gently decrease hyperventilation.

The Alexander Technique

This concentrates on achieving correct posture, which is often forgotten by both patient and therapist. Sufferers become aware of misusing muscles and can then correct bad posture habits, to benefit the whole body function.

Yoga

Yoga not only provides beneficial exercises for the body, but also teaches Pranayama breathing, which involves inhalation, exhalation, internal and external retention of breath. The fourth step, breathing out and holding the breath to different degrees, is similar but not identical to the Buteyko method.

Negative Ion Therapy

This therapy causes dust, pollutants and pollens to settle out from the air by negative and positive electronic attraction, so they cease being irritants to the respiratory system. Positive ions (electrically charged molecules) attract dust, smoke and pollens, and the negative-ion generator causes them to be quickly and effectively cleared from the air.

Massage and Aromatherapy

These therapies provide deep emotional and physical relaxation. Other benefits of massage include the improvement of circulation, clearing the lymphatic systems, and relaxation and toning-up of muscles and tendons.

When aromatherapy is used, these actions are enhanced by the use of essential oils from aromatic plants that have healing scents. The very part of the brain that houses our emotions also contains our scent receptors. Thus our perception of different scents is intertwined with our emotions and sense of well-being. Two useful plant scents are lavender, which has a relaxing effect, and eucalyptus, which is antiseptic and helps to clear mucus.

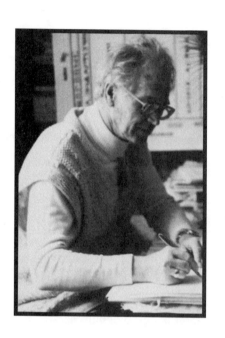

The Buteyko Method in Russia

Konstantin Buteyko's Medical Training

Konstantin Pavlovich Buteyko was born into a peasant family in 1923, in the village of Ivanitsa, near Kiev in Russia. His father was an enthusiast about anything mechanical and he passed his interests on to his son. After his schooling Buteyko began studies at the Kiev Polytechnic Institute. But these were interrupted by World War II, when he served in the Russian military forces. After the war his interest took a humanistic turn and he enrolled in the First Medical Institute in Moscow. He was then 23 years old.

Buteyko was hoping he would be able to diagnose medical problems in much the same way as he fixed machinery during the war — but medicine turned out to be more complex and more fascinating than he had imagined.

In his third year of medical studies, Buteyko was active in the clinical therapy group, supervised by the academic

OPPOSITE PAGE: *Professor Konstantin Buteyko in his laboratory.*

head of the department, Evengly Mikhailovitch Tareiev. After graduating from the Institute with honours in 1952, Buteyko became a clinical therapy intern in the same group, and was given the task of establishing a functional diagnostics laboratory in Moscow.

In 1958, Buteyko was invited by Professor Meshalkin to join the Institute of Experimental Biology and Medicine at the Siberian Branch of the USSR Academy of Science, where Meshalkin was director. The invitation was for the purpose of establishing a laboratory of functional diag-nostics. The project was to be completed in 1960.

Research into Deep Breathing

Buteyko's destiny was decided when he became involved in an independent practical assignment for his third year of medical studies. For this, he was asked to work out a method of auscultation (listening with a stethoscope) and he spent hundreds of hours listening to the breathing of patients.

One day, when he asked a patient to breathe deeply, the patient fainted. Buteyko was concerned, and in dis-cussion with others was told this was due to oxygen oversaturation of the brain. The patient's strong reaction to heavy breathing continued to intrigue him, however. Then, one night in the midst of the second month of his research, he came up with an entirely new concept —

that certain diseases might develop as a result of deep breathing. He had a ready patient to experiment on — himself. His own health problem was hypertension: in fact he was diagnosed as having malignant hypertension, the most severe form of high blood pressure.

He experimented by reducing his breathing: he noticed immediately that the headache he was suffering from at the time was reduced, and his rapid pulse slowed down. As soon as he increased the depth of his breathing, the symptoms returned. He was convinced he was on the way to discovering the cause of his disease.

He decided it was fair to presume that if deep breathing could cause the blood vessel spasm that occurred in hypertension, it could also produce the symptoms of other diseases. That night he stayed on at the clinic, checking and rechecking this idea on his patients.

Buteyko asked asthmatics to breathe more shallowly and their attacks stopped. He asked patients with chest pain, suffering from angina pectoris, to breathe more shallowly, and their attacks also stopped. Whenever these patients breathed more deeply, their attacks resumed.

By the very next morning, Buteyko was convinced that he had made a major discovery. He also realised that the medicine he had been studying was all upside-down. How could this be? For another month, he searched intensively for information to clear up the question — was it possible that, in the whole field of medical science, such a simple thought had never occurred to anyone else?

During his search, he learned of some experiments

which seemed to support his thinking, but just the same no one had actually tried to reduce breathing in their patients and record the results, or draw any conclusions from this. For centuries, the human race had been learning that it was healthy to breathe deeply.

Sharing the Results of Research

Buteyko then decided to share his thoughts — but he got no support from his teachers or his colleagues. He was discouraged, but not surprised. After all, he was not alone in striking scepticism and lack of cooperation from traditional medicine, when trying to promulgate a new idea. There were two good examples of this in the nineteenth century.

Semmelweiss in Hungary and Lister in England had each had similar problems in getting colleagues to listen to a new medical discovery. Semmelweiss in 1846 and Lister in 1867 each came to the conclusion that cross-infection of diseases from one patient to another could occur during medical treatment, and that using disinfectants and washing hands could help doctors reduce it. During their time it was normal to lose one-third of patients after surgery or after delivery of a baby, due to infection. It was also generally accepted medical practice to dissect bodies at post mortem examinations and then to carry out such things as surgery without any hygiene precautions at all.

Semmelweiss tested and confirmed his own theory by setting up a three-month trial where patients were given fresh sheets on the beds, and antiseptics were used to wash the hands of medical staff. He lost no patients at all from infection in those three months. He continued to use and promote these hygiene methods, but such was the backlash against him that he was eventually declared to be mentally disturbed. He was committed to a mental asylum, and in time he died there. In England, the same hygiene practices were championed by Lister, but it was only when the discovery actually reached the ears of the general public that it gained recognition. Patients' relatives started to turn up at hospitals before operations, demanding to know whether surgeons at the hospitals were washing their hands before touching patients. Only then did the procedure become accepted by physicians — 50 years after Semmelweiss's initial discovery.

Buteyko understood, then, that simply voicing his convictions would not necessarily convince his colleagues: he would have to gather evidence, develop it, find a formula to express the fundamentals of his idea — then announce it. He needed an experimental laboratory.

Buteyko's Clinical Studies

Fortunately the establishment of the functional diagnostics laboratory at Professor Meshalkin's Institute in Siberia could be carried out alongside Buteyko's own work. In 1958–59, clinical studies were conducted on the breathing and the condition of about 200 people, both healthy and sick. Buteyko could now show studies which scientifically confirmed the correctness of his discovery.

On 11 January 1960, Buteyko presented his work to the Scientific Forum at the Institute and explained the basis of his thinking. He described his experiments, which showed the objective interdependence between depth of breathing (hyperventilation), the content of carbon dioxide in the human body, vessel spasms in the patients studied, and the condition of their health.

Most of the members were stunned. Buteyko was suggesting that such diseases such as asthma, hypertension and angina pectoris could be cured without a knife. Buteyko had expected that this would be welcome news, for everybody knew that invasive surgery never cured these diseases and mortality from them was high. But Buteyko's suggested cure, founded on shallow breathing, got a very muted response.

Despite this lack of enthusiasm amongst Buteyko's colleagues, however, Professor Meshalkin, who had chaired the forum, gave his approval for the research to continue. Using the best scientific and technological means available at the time, extensive information was obtained on the basic functions of the human organism, whether healthy or diseased. The information was analysed on computers which mathematically derived physiological measurements and various conclusions from the figures.

Two hundred specialists were being trained in the laboratory, and they also took part, for most of whom suffered one condition or another and could try the method on themselves before they treated other patients. *Statistics available from Russia show that by 1967, more than 1,000 patients suffering from asthma, hypertension or angina had been successfully treated with the method and had totally recovered from their illnesses.*

Professor Meshalkin himself consulted Buteyko about his own heart condition. Tests were conducted, and Meshalkin was found to be in imminent danger of a serious heart attack. Within a few days of using the breathing method, his health improved. Nevertheless, when Buteyko requested official approval of the method, Professor Meshalkin vetoed it.

Subsequently Buteyko was told that there were to be no publications, public appearances or speeches made on the subject of his work. This prohibition reflected the attitude shared by Meshalkin and his student surgeons. Later, equipment was confiscated from the laboratory and the Institute laboratory was disbanded and closed. Buteyko, however, was able to keep one third of all the instruments, personnel and premises.

Meshalkin's clinic was eventually assimilated into the system of the Ministry of Health of the USSR (now Russia). From 1963–1968 Buteyko's own laboratory became attached to the Institute of Cytology and Genetics of the Siberian Branch of the USSR Academy of Science. Even in this new situation, his repeated requests to do research, and attempts to use experimentation to accredit the method, failed completely.

In January 1968, representations were made by local and foreign press in defence of his discovery, and at last approbation was carried out in Leningrad, at the Institute of Pulmonology. The Minister of Health informed Buteyko that if he successfully treated at least 80% of his patients, the minister would make recommendations for an immediate inclusion of the method into medical practice in Russia. He also promised the use of a 50-bed clinic for the continuation of the clinical work. There was a condition — Buteyko would have to accept the most serious and difficult cases that were not otherwise treatable by conventional, medical methods. Within a short time, 44 of Buteyko's 46 patients were officially recognised as cured and, after further treatment, the remaining two also recovered. Consequently the results of the method in this case could be described as having a 100% success rate.

There was another twist of fate (or officialdom) lying in wait for Buteyko, however. The official conclusions of the approbation were sent to the Health Minister but were never made known to Buteyko, nor to the Siberian Branch of the Academy of Science. Later, the Ministry advised that the approbation had failed, stating that only two of the 46 patients had been cured. Next, this falsification of the findings was used as an excuse for closing the laboratory. On 14 August 1968, Buteyko's laboratory was closed and his personnel dismissed without offers of alternative employment. All his equipment was confiscated.

Acceptance of the Buteyko Method in Russia

Despite this catastrophe, the Buteyko Method survived, because the teams of medicos Buteyko had trained in his clinic continued to treat patients. Over the years, the news of their successes forced the government to review the method. The second official approbation was conducted at the First Moscow Institute of Paediatric Diseases in April 1980. *The study confirmed the results of the earlier approbation, which by then had become public, through word of mouth and press reports. The Russian summaries, which I have read in translation, show that the method as practised by all patients had a 100% success rate in treating their condition.* The results were officially recognised, and the Buteyko Method is now endorsed by the Russian government.

Professor Buteyko continues to work as a respiratory physician and to treat patients for asthma, and has established himself in Novosibirsk. At the age of 74 (in 1997) he travels between Moscow and Novosibirsk, lecturing on his research, treating patients, and tutoring practitioners in the Buteyko method. This outspoken, authoritative and colourful man is a household name in Russia, where people know him from his work, and from the press, television and videos. His method is now poised to help millions around the world.

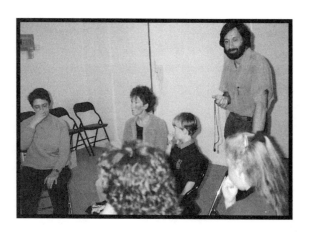

The Buteyko Method in Other Countries

Australia

The first practitioner of the Buteyko method in Australia was a Russian, Alexander Stalmatsky (known as Sasha), who had studied under Professor Buteyko for 14 years. He was very aware of the fact that Australia and New Zealand have per capita more asthma sufferers than anywhere in the world, and this influenced his choice of a new country in which to practise.

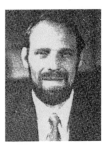

Alexander Stalmatsky (Sasha)

Sasha arrived in Sydney in October 1990. From a humble one-bedroom flat in Bondi Junction, and with limited knowledge of English, Sasha nonetheless began to treat patients. He started with Russian friends who suffered variously from asthma, emphysema, blood pressure, sinusitis, stress/anxiety syndrome and obesity.

OPPOSITE PAGE: *The author conducts a Buteyko class in a country clinic.*

Word started to spread, and more and more people benefited from the method. I first learned of it when two patients, a mother and a daughter, came to my practice and informed me that there was a new breathing technique which they had participated in. Following the exercise regime, the mother was able to stop medical treatment altogether, and her daughter reduced her previous treatment to half (she was somewhat resistant at first to carrying out the exercises, being an active and busy teenager).

I decided to ring and find out more about this technique.

The Buteyko group was moving to Edgecliff, I was told, and Sasha had teamed up with a resourceful young man called Christopher Drake. Christopher's background was in health-related business: he had previously helped set up chains of cellulite treatment clinics, and he had experience with European Health Rejuvenation Clinics. These experiences had whetted his appetite to promote a completely holistic health treatment, and he was impressed with Buteyko's method with its 90%-plus effectiveness. He saw this as an opportunity to put his hard-earned abilities behind a method that was an effective treatment and not a cosmetic improvement to people's well-being.

Convinced, by what he witnessed, of the enormous importance of Buteyko's discovery, he set out to make the technique known to the public and the medical world. His awesome energy and marketing expertise soon placed the Buteyko Method on the map.

Working to a phenomenal schedule, Buteyko workshops were quickly set up in all the states' capital cities.

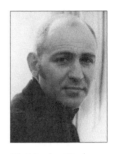

Christopher Drake

Invitations to refer patients on to the workshops were sent out to G.P.s, specialists and naturopathic practitioners. Very soon, one respiratory specialist attended a workshop, and two other respiratory specialists referred some patients.

As patient numbers swelled, it became clear that more teachers would be needed, and training of new teachers was offered as a franchise. Improved patients, naturopaths and one G.P., Dr Kevin Tracey (who had treated himself by using the method), took up the opportunity. As of July 1995, there were some 24 trained practitioners in Australia. Word of mouth soon swelled the numbers of patients further.

When I appeared on television for the first time to comment on the technique, however, I found that I was the only doctor in Australia who recommended it. News about the method began to feature in most newspapers and magazines, including the *Sun Herald*, *The Daily Telegraph*, *The Bulletin*, *Natural Health Society* magazine, *Wellbeing*, *Health and Nature* etc. Television reports that featured Buteyko were the *7.30 Report*, *A Current Affair*, *Real Life*, the *Today*, *Tonight Show* and news broadcasts from various channels.

The technique also reached rural areas. The first workshop in country areas was in Mudgee in August 1994, the instructors being Christopher Drake and the author. Other country practitioners in 1997 included Gregory Parnell.

In December 1994, the Australian Buteyko Association was formed. The meetings were held at the Vita Centre in Edgecliff, Sydney, under chairperson Rosalba Belford, a naturopath who is also a practitioner of the Buteyko method. She led the two-day meeting of 16 Buteyko teachers, other therapists and some patients. The purpose of the meeting was to settle on a Constitution and to form a Code of Ethics. It was decided that a membership fee would be charged, and the funds would be used to gain resources to carry out general meetings every three months. A list of all practitioners in Australia and their contact details was drawn up, and is kept updated by the Association.

The First Scientific, Clinical Trial of Buteyko in the Western World

When the Buteyko method became better known in Australia, the Asthma Foundations were heavily pressured by the media to respond, and hundreds of cured patients rang the Foundations to ask them to take note of their experiences of cure.

The Australian Asthma Foundations could not of course recommend the method themselves at that point, as there had not been any clinical scientific trial carried out in Australia or the Western world. Their impression was that all they had as information was one doctor crying out 'from the wilderness' and hundreds of people with 'anecdotes' about the method, who were swearing that they could control their asthma, and talking about how the method had changed their lives.

BUTEYKO TREATMENT FOR ASTHMA

There has been recent television and other publicity implying that the Buteyko treatment is a new development. The following article appeared in the Foundation's June 1992 newsletter.

WARNING – ON POTENTIALLY DANGEROUS ASTHMA TREATMENT

The Asthma Foundation of Victoria has issued a public warning to asthmatics about BUTEYKO treatment. This follows recent media exposure of this treatment being introduced in Australia.

The Asthma Foundation of Victoria does not recommend the Buteyko method for the treatment of asthma.

The available literature on the Buteyko method has been examined by the Asthma Foundation. Most of this literature emanates from the USSR. It particularly relates to hypoxitherapy and volitional respiration.

1. Hypoxitherapy
The proposed procedure is dangerous and it is doubtful if any institutional ethics committee would allow it to be part of any research project dealing with humans.

2. Volitional Respiration
It is possible that elevated carbon dioxide levels may relax bronchial muscle tone and thus relieve some symptoms in acute asthma. However, using elevated carbon dioxide levels in treatment would need specialised knowledge and its potential dangers to be fully recognised.

Any benefit from training in volitional respiration would derive from an increased awareness of relaxed breathing. The benefits of correcting hyperventilation and promoting slow breathing have long been recognised. They are, however, dwarfed by benefits of pharmaceutical therapy.

Since the benefits from volitional respiration would be minor, there is a risk if it is promoted as a major advance in asthma therapy. It is basically psychotherapy and the Foundation rejects the physiological basis claimed for it.

This Foundation believes it would be in the public interest for the promoters of this method to be identified and their medical advisors also to be disclosed.

A facsimile of the warning issued by the Asthma Foundation of Victoria before the Queensland trial.

Initially, the Victorian Asthma Foundation actually released a pamphlet warning sufferers that the method was unproven and telling them to be wary of it. This nearly resulted in the Buteyko organisation bringing a legal suit against the Victorian Asthma Foundation, but they contained themselves. They decided instead to work more determinedly to establish some Australian research.

Even though one million patients had undergone Buteyko training in the clinics in Russia, and there was a sample of 100,000 cures officially documented by Professor Buteyko, and even though there were rooms full of research materials available from Russia (volumes about the above research, already translated into English) no one capable of undertaking research into asthma in Australia seemed interested in setting up scientific trials into the method.

Finally it was decided to carry out a preliminary open clinical trial in Victoria, to investigate this Russian Approach. A few details concerning the method in Russia struck some observers in Australia as outlandish. For instance, sea salt is sometimes used orally during Buteyko classes to enhance the breathing technique. Some patients in Russia (but not Buteyko patients) actually used to be placed in rooms hollowed out from solid salt walls — in this situation, their breathing improved noticeably. This information led to all sorts of remarks about Russian salt mines! But there is no connection between this method and Buteyko. The Asthma Foundations were invited to send observers to the proposed trial, but did not do so. By contrast, a Buteyko trial in February 1994 was observed by the Asthma Foundation in Adelaide.

The Victorian open trial did take place, however, with a group of asthma sufferers following the Buteyko technique. One week after the trial began, the group were performing significantly better in managing their asthma.

Then followed the Queensland trial, which was a

closed, scientific trial. In the lead-up time, there was prolonged but civil to-and-fro communication between the
Buteyko group and the Queensland University team.
Finally an agreement was reached for a controlled, randomised trial of the Buteyko technique. The trial was supported by a grant from the Australian Association of
Asthma Foundations. This was a planned, two-centre,
three-month study on 40 subjects — these were all people who had asthma that was being treated with well-
documented and significant bronchodilator use.

The Results of the Queensland Trial
The Queensland team consisted of Associate Professor
Charles Mitchell, Dr Simon Bowler and Ms Amanda Green.
The BB (Buteyko) team consisted of Sasha Stalmatsky and
Ms Tess Graham.

After a four-week run-in phase, subjects were strati-
fied on the basis of bronchodilator and steroid use and
grouped evenly according to age, sex etc. (randomised).
Nineteen went to Buteyko Breathing (BB) classes for 90
minutes a day for one week. For the same period, the 20
others, who did not do the method, were given as much
help from current medical practice as could be provided,
such as physiotherapy classes (PC), standard asthma education, breathing and coughing and relaxation exercises.

After six weeks, the results of the trial up to that point
were set out in a report. Here is a quote from the report:

*At six weeks, after learning Buteyko breathing exercises,
each member of a group of 19 patients with moderately severe*

asthma was able to reduce his or her use of relieving medication (Ventolin, Bricanyl etc.) by 90%. A similar group of 20 patients who received general advice about asthma and some simple stress techniques enjoyed no such improvement.

5% reduction in medication was the best that the control group could achieve.

Doctors gasp at Buteyko success

BUTEYKO breathing hypoventilation exercises in patients with asthma reduced beta agonist use by 90% and improved symptoms, according to preliminary results of a randomised, controlled trial in Brisbane.

However, there were no changes in major physiological parameters such as peak flow rate or FEV_1 in people using Buteyko breathing.

The study was reported at a meeting of the Thoracic Society of Australia and New Zealand in Hobart last week by Dr Simon Bowler, a respiratory physician at Mater Hospital in Brisbane.

Dr Bowler said there were no obvious explanations for the apparent short-term benefits of Buteyko breathing.

"We were surprised at the results, as we didn't expect any significant changes," he told Australian Doctor.

Proponents of the technique claimed that hypoventilation and the subsequent increase in carbon dioxide levels could relieve the symptoms of bronchospasm and favourably affect the long-term course of asthma.

The study was prompted by publicity about Buteyko breathing and the number of inquiries to asthma foundations and requests for advice from other health professionals it had generated.

The study was funded by the Australian Association of Asthma Foundations. Forty patients with well-documented asthma and significant daily use of bronchodilators were recruited and randomised to a Buteyko or control group — 39 remained in the study.

The Buteyko group received classes from a Buteyko practitioner for 90 minutes a day for seven days and the classes included direct encouragement to minimise beta agonist use.

The control patients received a similar regimen of physiotherapy classes which included standard asthma education, breathing exercises (excluding any hypoventilation) and relaxation techniques. Both groups were carefully instructed to use bronchodilators only as required and not on a routine basis.

"We would expect education to influence the patients' asthma management, but wouldn't normally expect the other techniques to have any major effect on medication use or respiratory function," Dr Bowler said.

"After six weeks there was a 90% reduction in beta agonist use in the Buteyko group, compared to only a 5% reduction in the control group."

There was also a significant difference in quality of life and improvement in symptom scores in the Buteyko group.

"These changes occurred in the absence of any
cont'd page 2

All the results up to that point in the trial were released on March 30, 1995 at the Annual Scientific Meeting of the Thoracic Society of Australia and New Zealand, in Hobart. Five hundred leading respiratory medicine specialists and researchers from around Australia and New Zealand attended this conference at Hobart's West Point Convention Centre. It was a significant exposure of the method to an important, influential collection of scientific minds. In addition, a surge of public and media response resulted.

The second half of the three-month assessment was still to come, but people were already excited. Articles appeared in regional newspapers and in health magazines, and for the first time in the *Australian Doctor* (front page story) and *Medical Observer*, and there were letters in the *Medical Journal of Australia*. This surge of interest was one of the things that stimulated me to begin writing this book: I realised that people were demanding information, and it was time

from page 1

improvement in airflow," Dr Bowler said.

"In this study, there appears to be some short-term benefit from Buteyko techniques in terms of reduced beta agonist use, without obvious cost in terms of worsening symptom scores."

The trial continued for another six weeks to investigate the effect of reducing inhaled corticosteroid use, but the data are yet to be analysed.

— Tony James

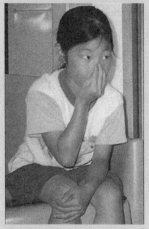

A child with asthma practises breath holding at a Buteyko method workshop.

An article from Australian Doctor, 7 April 1995

learned about the method so they could judge for themselves. Here is part of a press release at that time.

'Buteyko practitioners have been enthusiastic about the value of the exercises, though the orthodox medical community has been sceptical,' said Dr Bowler, representing the University of Queensland researchers.

'Professor Buteyko's theories, whilst interesting, are not supported by any published scientific data in the Western literature and we have only had case reports of success to go on until now.'

Dr Bowler then mentioned the results above — 90% reduction in bronchodilator use by the Buteyko patients. He went on:

'In addition, measures of how the subjects were feeling showed a greater benefit from the Buteyko technique. Both groups of subjects were initially found to have high ventilation rates and low breath carbon dioxide levels,' said Dr Bowler. 'In the Buteyko group, ventilation fell by about 30% with a trend towards higher CO_2 levels. No such change occurred in the standard treatment group.'

The University researchers say they are cautious about drawing too strong a conclusion from the preliminary data.

'The results suggest an immediate benefit from Buteyko although there were no changes in test of airway calibre,' explained Dr Mitchell.

'That is, asthmatics in the Buteyko group felt better, and used less bronchodilating medicine, but the narrowing of

Buteyko lowers need for drug

PATIENTS with asthma using the Buteyko technique to decrease their breathing volumes reduced their inhaled corticosteroid use by 30%, a Brisbane trial has found.

Preliminary results of the study released last year showed a 90% drop in the use of beta agonist bronchodilators in people using the technique.

However, researchers involved in the trial contacted by *Australian Doctor* disagreed over the implications of the results.

The trial, conducted at the Mater Hospital, randomised 39 adults with longstanding asthma to 90-minute Buteyko classes daily for seven days, or a similar regimen of standard physiotherapy classes.

The researchers, including respiratory physician Dr Simon Bowler, monitored medication use and respiratory function in the next 12 weeks.

Steroid use was regulated by doctors using a protocol based on patients' prn use of bronchodilators.

Dr Bowler said the study showed Buteyko was a useful technique for assisting patients with asthma.

"But from the trial and subsequent experience with other patients, I don't believe that it improves lung function and I don't think it necessarily alters the underlying asthma," he said.

"It does, though, seem to improve the interaction between patients and their asthma, allowing a better sense of control and mastery.

"There is a group in whom it's extremely useful — those who have excess dependence on beta agonists."

Dr Bowler said this was just one study and it needed to be repeated.

"Just as no operative technique or drug would be accepted on the basis of one trial, the Buteyko method needs to be further investigated."

Tess Graham, the Buteyko practitioner who trained the patients in the trial, criticised the conclusion that the underlying disease was not affected.

She said the study showed Buteyko techniques reduced the over-breathing claimed to be the basis of asthma.

"There are now solid grounds for thinking that many of the 800 asthma sufferers and 6000 with sleep apnoea who die each year in Australia could be saved by applying the techniques of Dr Konstantin Buteyko," she said.

— Tony James

Also from Australian Doctor.

their bronchial tubes did not improve.

'Furthermore, we have only analysed the data from the six-week assessment. We are now conducting the three-month evaluation, assessing the usefulness of the technique in reducing the amount of preventative medication (e.g. Becotide, Becloforte, Pulmicort) needed,' Dr Mitchell said.

Since then, the results of the full three-month assessment have been written up, and are available. But they have not yet been published by the *Medical Journal of Australia* or released to the medical profession. We know however that the Buteyko patients came out of the six-week trial with airways similar to those of the 'control' group, but in contrast to the others they were breathing more easily and were free of symptoms while continuing with very little bronchodilator use, and in some cases no use of drugs at all.

The increasing desire for knowledge about this important study will no doubt lead to publication of the full trial results. The response to the Buteyko method continues to grow in Australia. In 1997 there were around 40 practitioners. A group of patients also formed a lobby group in 1995 to promote the Buteyko technique in Australia. Dr Ian Brighthope, the president of the Australian College of Nutritional and Environmental Medicine (ACNEM), invited the author to lecture about nutrition and Buteyko at the first ACNEM educational meeting in Sydney in May 1996. I spoke to some 45 doctors, dentists and pharmacists. The Australian Medical Acupuncture Society (AMAS) has also asked me to lecture about Buteyko. Buteyko is a method eminently compatible with many Eastern practices: for instance, breathing exercises play a large part in Chinese medicine, e.g. Chi Gong, Tai Chi.

The results of the first clinical trial of the Buteyko method conducted in Australia are couched in medical terms not easily accessible to the general reader, but here we have included a table (opposite) giving some of the results. They show reduction of bronchodilator use and substantial reduction of inhaled steroid use, over a period of time, by the Buteyko (BBT) group during the trial.

DAILY BRONCHODILATOR USE

Total for 19 Patients	5/12/94 Pre Instruction	13/12/94	22/12/94 10 Days Post Instruction	9/1/95 5 Weeks Post Instruction
Atrovent puffs	13	0	0	0
Atrovent nebulisers	11 ½	0	0	0
Ventolin puffs	123	8	10	8–10
Ventolin nebulisers	14	1 ½	½	0–½
Bricanyl puffs	4	0	1	0
Bricanyl nebulisers	2	0	0	0
Serevent puffs	12	11	10	3
Theodur mg	2300	600	600	600
Aostyn mg	900	900	300	300
Elixophyllin ml	60	40	30	?

Profile Patient (No 16)				
Ventolin puffs	8	4	0–6	1–2
Ventolin nebuliser	4	1	½–1	0–½
Atrovent nebuliser	4	0	0	0
Theodur mg	500	600	600	600
Pulmicort puffs	12	12	12	12
Intal puffs	8	8	8	8
Prednisone mg	0	0	30	10

New Zealand

New Zealand has the highest incidence of asthma in the world. It is estimated that approximately 700,000 people, or 20% of the population, have this condition. In 1995 one in five children and one in three Maori were told they had asthma.

In New Zealand as in other countries, asthma drugs are a very big business; they are among the most expensive, costing the New Zealand Regional Health Authorities $112 million in the year to June 1995. In that year 687,000 preventer-type inhalers — often cortico-steroids — were sold, and 1,521,000 reliever-type inhalers, such as Ventolin. Hospital care for asthmatics alone costs $23 million per year (1997 figures), as much as for heart surgery.

Buteyko has been taught in New Zealand since January 1994 by Russell and Jennifer Stark, who hold courses or workshops spread over six consecutive days in all major towns throughout the country. To date they have taught some 2500 asthmatics to take better control over their asthma while using less drug medication.

The New Zealand Asthma and Respiratory Foundation is not opposed to Buteyko, according to Executive Director, Sarah Thompson, and Medical Director, Dr Julian Crane. They recommend that if large changes to drug regimes are to be made by patients then consultation with their doctor is a must. This is in accordance with the Starks' own recommendation. They make it very clear throughout every course that asthmatics use reliever medication when it is necessary and they must consult their doctor before reducing preventive medication.

In 1995 Dr Julian Crane stated in a report to the New Zealand Asthma Societies:

(1) There is no scientific evidence yet available to assess the effectiveness of Buteyko in asthma.

(2) There do not appear to be any obvious problems with safety and the advice given by Buteyko to use 'relievers' when required and continue with 'preventers' is in accord with current medical advice.

(3) Individuals planning to try the technique should inform and discuss their intentions with their doctor especially if they are contemplating changes to their treatment.

Since that time, further correspondence and a meeting has been held between Buteyko and the Directors of the Asthma and Respiratory Foundation, and research was being discussed in 1997.

The Asthma Societies throughout New Zealand can have differing approaches from the Asthma and Respiratory Foundation. The Societies are usually run by volunteers and paid asthma educators. Depending on how Dr Julian Crane's statement has been interpreted by staff and volunteers, people inquiring about the technique may be given advice ranging from, 'You have nothing to lose,' to, 'We teach the same exercises ourselves for free. Don't enrol.' Some have got behind Buteyko and encourage people to learn the method.

Perhaps because of the rather conciliatory attitude of the New Zealand Asthma and Respiratory Foundation and the medical profession as a whole, no controversy has taken place between Buteyko New Zealand, their supporters, and those advocating conventional asthma therapies. This has meant that Buteyko, although it is a drug-free method, has attracted little media interest, and the Starks have therefore had to rely on 'word of mouth' and their own advertising skills to promote the technique.

When people first hear about Buteyko, scepticism can still be a major problem in New Zealand. Because asthma symptoms and triggers are so varied, asthmatics have a tendency to think that a Buteyko course 'might help others but it won't help me.' Many New Zealanders have previously tried physiotherapy breathing exercises for asthma, with little success, and so are not willing to try something which they consider similar.

Cost and availability of the courses can also be a problem for some asthmatics. Buteyko courses are also only available at certain times of the year in each New Zealand town. Therefore, the Starks encourage some sufferers to learn the technique first and then pay off the course fees as they can afford, over a period of time.

Russell Stark has addressed health professionals such as doctors, nurses, physiotherapists, asthma educators and natural therapists at various forums. He has spoken at the Asthma/CORD link in 1995, the South Pacific Association of Natural Therapists in 1996 and the South Island Respiratory Educators Forum in 1997. Buteyko New Zealand has also held two seminars specifically for health professionals in Wellington and Hastings.

Some naturopaths, chiropractors and physiotherapists regularly recommend the method to their patients, as do a number of GPs and respiratory specialists throughout the country. The Starks have taught the Buteyko method to several family members of doctors and through this, as well as the observations of their own patients who have attended the courses, credibility is growing.

People intending to learn the technique are invited to bring their doctor with them. Any interested health professional is encouraged to attend at least the first and last sessions of a course to see for him or herself how the method works and monitor the results after it has been practised for a few days.

The United Kingdom

Statistics from 1997 show that one in 20 British adults suffers from asthma, and in the UK it causes seven million days off work and kills someone every four hours. Asthma prescriptions cost the National Health Service £350 million a year (a figure which doubled in ten years).

The first practitioners of the Buteyko method in England were Christopher Drake and Alexander Stalmatsky. Christopher Drake went to England in 1994 and commenced practice at French Medical Centre in South Kensington. One of the patients he treated was Mr Jonathan Aitken, then Treasury Chief Secretary. His asthma was moderately severe, but over a course of consultations and home visits he made a dramatic recovery.

Jonathan Aitken said in a newspaper article: 'I have tried plenty of treatments, but this is the only one that has really worked. I think it is a remarkable one that could help many people.' He also remarked that the news of the 'simple and natural' Buteyko method might 'ruffle the feathers of the drug manufacturers', but he emphasised that for asthma sufferers the big question was: 'Does it work or not?' He concluded: 'It did for me.'

These remarks were made in a full-page *Daily Mail* article by Jessica Fisher, entitled 'Member of Parliament Backs Method'. Another *Daily Mail* article which included an interview with Christopher Drake had the headline, 'Could this be the end of the Inhaler?'. As a result of other articles and publicity, he received thousands of inquiries from all over the country and proceeded to hold workshops in London, Birmingham, Glasgow, Manchester and other cities and towns. Eventually he moved the practice to Number 12 Harley Street, where he held consultations and conducted workshops.

Major newspapers and periodicals in the UK which have featured the Buteyko method are: the *Independent*, *Daily Mail*, *Daily Express*, *Herald*, the *Scotsman*, *Irish Times*, *Harpers* and *Queen*.

Christopher has also featured on many television documentaries and radio shows. Following some of his remarks about the benefits of the method on a BBC2 documentary, where he also talked about traditional approaches to asthma, he was for a time under threat of legal action by the National Asthma Campaign.

He has a characteristically graphic way of helping people understand the Buteyko theory that is outlined in this book. He says: 'Asthmatics are chronically hyperventilating all the time. Imagine if our body temperature was five times what it should be: we'd be dead. Well, some asthmatics breathe five times more than they should.' He explains the importance of carbon dioxide in the body by calling it 'the body's own bronchodilator'. As he points out, the Buteyko method is simple, but it takes commitment to change the breathing habits of a lifetime and learn to breathe for one person. He stresses that the method is quite safe, as medication is only reduced as people's symptoms improve. 'The breathing technique acts like Ventolin, as a bronchodilator. You only take headache tablets if you have a headache. If you don't have bronchospasm, why take a bronchodilator?'

In 1997 Christopher Drake was spending time equally between London and a second Buteyko practice that he established in Dublin, Ireland.

Buteyko in the USA

Aaron Lumsdaine of Perth, Australia, has never suffered from asthma, but he first realised its frightening dangers in 1989 when the mother of a close friend died as the result of an attack. The funeral of this 43-year-old woman was attended by 400 people. She was the wife of a pharmacist and mother of two, who had followed the best medical advice and taken her medications as instructed. Yet she died from a heart attack induced by an asthma attack, at three o'clock in the morning, in the ambulance on the way to hospital.

At the time it appeared to Aaron that the death of this woman, who had helped and touched so many, was a senseless waste. But it was one of the things which made him investigate the Buteyko method a few years later, in Sydney. There he met with Jac Vidgen, the Marketing Manager for Buteyko Australia, Christopher Drake, and Russian Buteyko Practitioner Alexander Stalmatsky.

Once Aaron understood the efficacy of the method he returned to Perth determined that more people should have access to the benefits of the method.

He remembers: 'Everyone I spoke to said I was crazy. Why give up a perfectly sound management career with a major West Australian corporation to teach a 50-year-old Russian Breathing Technique?

'Three days to decide. The first time in my life I truly listened to my heart. Back I went, following the Russian around Australia learning how to become a Buteyko Practitioner.

'Collectively we taught around 200 people from Melbourne to Caloundra with many conditions, all with the same successes of reduced reliance on medication, greater energy levels, improved quality of life. People with epilepsy, emphysema, heart conditions, migraines and the list went on.

'Finally I qualified and back to Perth I came, establishing Buteyko Perth, WA in 1994. Since then I have taught over 1,000 people for a variety of conditions. They have been of all ages, all walks of life, and my clientele has included doctors, naturopaths, chiropractors, physiotherapists, nurses, psychiatrists, respiratory nurses, teachers, business people, sports people.'

In 1996 Buteyko practitioners from around Australia gathered and formed the non-profit Buteyko Institute for Breathing and Health Incorporated. As one of the Senior Buteyko Practitioners in Australia, Aaron was elected Executive Officer. The mission statement — to improve health by correcting asthma and other breathing-related disorders through research, development, promotion and application of the Buteyko Technique of Breathing Reconditioning.

His dream had always been to go to America, and on 4 January 1997 a plea came via Email for a Buteyko Practitioner to go to the USA to help a woman who had nearly died from an asthma attack. A few media releases went out to say Aaron was arriving, and by 17 February he was in Pennsylvania, explaining the physiology behind the Buteyko Technique and letting people know that there was a revolutionary treatment of asthma available. His introductory presentations were held at the Eressea Learning Center in Kempton, the Weller Center for Health in Easton, and the Academy of the NEW Church College Social Center in Bryn Athyn, PA, which all kindly donated the use of their facilities. Of the 59 people who attended these presentations, 17 were able to take the five-day course Aaron offered. Ages ranged from 5 to 74; conditions included asthma, migraines, allergies, hypoglycaemia, Chronic Fatigue Syndrome.

Patricia Odhner, the patient whose plight initially prompted Aaron to go to the USA, has this to say: 'I have been truly touched by everyone's concern. I feel wonderful! I continue to improve every day. I work at the exercises, yes, but it's worth it to find all those allergies slipping away — to discover I can smell again. Flowers! Spring! Snow! Air! And with no fear. NO MORE FEAR. Incredible!'

Below are brief stories of other people who have taken the Buteyko Course in the USA. Each would recommend the course to any asthmatic, and has given permission for their statement to be printed.

Gloria Schecter, Hamburg, PA, former asthma sufferer: 'I feel wonderful, I'm feeling great. I can't believe it. I'm off medication. I wish more people would look into it.'

Richard Heffner, Fleetwood, PA. Richard had asthma and emphysema with asbestos in his lungs. Now he is just about off medication and feels much better. He has more endurance and stamina. He has no more asthma symptoms. He says he would recommend the program for anyone.

Ginny Booth, Kempton, PA: 'Since I learned to use the Buteyko Method the quality of my life has changed significantly for the better. I'm resting well. My lungs are clearing up more every day. I have been able to stop taking theophylline for asthma after 12 years of daily use. It feels great to be in control of my breathing — and I no longer fear a trip to the emergency room.'

Guines Wiley-Nieves, a middle aged participant in the course, has had extremely serious asthma since his early youth. For three years running he has spent an average of one month in hospital each year. Since starting the Buteyko Breathing he has reduced the amount of inhaler (albuterol) by 50% or more. He says he is now confident that he will not end up in hospital any more.

Catherine Odhner, Huntingdon Valley, PA. Cathy was suffering from increasingly severe sinus headaches which sometimes lasted for several hours. She has not had a bad sinus headache since starting the course and has been able to use the breathing method to stop the headaches after 5–10 minutes when they arise.

Danielle Triplett, Easton, PA. Danielle, 12, had asthma, eczema, and perhaps of most concern, blackouts in which she would become very light-headed, dizzy, and lose her vision. In her karate class she would have to stop and take a breather (bronchodilator) before and after each sparring match, and got winded quickly. Since she started the Buteyko classes, Danielle's parents Joanne and Stan report that the blackouts have stopped. She had a few instances of blurring coming on but was able to prevent the blackouts when she did the breathing. One weekend she was able to spar for ten minutes and actually outlasted her opponent. Her eczema cleared up measurably, but she still has ups and downs.

Mabel Reader, Topton, PA. Mabel used to have an asthma attack about once a month. She has not had an attack since starting the Buteyko Method. She has stopped taking her 'breath air', her reliever medication, and has recently been able to spend all day outside which she could not have done before because her allergies would flare up and an asthma attack would follow.

Ira Rupp, Orefield, PA. Ira stated that before his Buteyko course he was so weak from asthma that he could hardly do anything. Most times he could only get halfway up the basement steps before having to rest. He now says that he has no need to stop for anything. He has cut his dose of reliever medication in half.

Caleb Kerr, Kempton, PA. In the last conversation with Aaron Lumsdaine, Caleb's mother Carla said Caleb, 9, was still congested but he was not doing his exercises as faithfully as prescribed and still breathing a lot through his mouth (a Buteyko transgression!). Nevertheless he had not had any wheeziness in quite a while and was no longer on bronchodilators.

Mathew and Brandon Brezezinski, Easton, PA. Mathew and Brandon are five-year-old twins. Their parents Louanne and Pete said that they are convinced that the method works but it is still difficult to get such young children to maintain the exercise regime. Both boys have reduced their need for bronchodilators. Allergies no longer seem to bother Mathew at a friend's house, which used to aggravate his asthma.

Paige Holm, Glenside, PA: 'I haven't had any medication since I started the classes. That's pretty much a miracle for me. I'm absolutely able to get rid of an asthma attack or wheeziness by doing the breathing. For anyone with asthma, it's definitely worth checking out. I'm not even hypoglycaemic any more — before I had to eat every two hours to keep my blood sugar up, now I need to eat a lot less.'

During his stay in the USA, Aaron established the non-profit Buteyko USA Ltd. In 1997 he had plans to hold sessions in other parts of the USA including Hawaii. Back in Australia he finished work on a Buteyko website and finalised the business plans for expansion throughout Western Australia, the Northern Territory, the USA and Canada.

Aaron now travels regularly between Australia and North America and is CEO of Buteyko USA Ltd.

⊕ **Бутейко Константин Павлович**

Автор метода ВЛГД (патент1067640,патент1593627),академик МАИ,кандидат медицинских наук
Президент Российской и Украинской Академий Спирокультуры,
генеральный директор и научный руководитель Ассоциации лечебно-оздоровительныхцентров
"Дыхание по Бутейко"
и Общества защиты открытий и изобретений Бутейко

111123 Россия,Москва,3-яВла- димирская ул.,д.3 корп.2 т304-18-89 176-00-63 306-47-50	Украина,Киев т.225-09-17 265-84-34 255-71-55	630090 Россия, Новосибирск ул.Жемчужная 4-19 т.35-09-19 32-02-81

24.02.96. Уважаемый доктор Paul Amaisen!

Я узнал о Вашей книге где вы рас-
казали о пользе моего метода лечения
астмы и некоторых других болезней
уменьшением глубины дыхания
запатентованым в России

(N 1067640 приорет от 29 янв. 1962г)

Благодарю Вас за понимание
сути моего открытия заклю-
чающегося в Гипервентиляции
как причина этих болезней.

Желаю Вам успеха в пропаганде
этого открытия, которое 44 год не
может достигнуть всех людей на
земле из-за консерватизма
медицины. с уважением

The letter to the author from Professor Buteyko, 24 February 1996.

Appendices

A Letter from Professor Buteyko
Translated from Russian

Dear Dr Paul Ameisen,

I am aware of your book in which you explain about the benefits of my method of treatment of asthma and some other diseases by decreasing the depth of breathing, patented in Russia (Patent 1067640 or 1593677, January 29, 1962).

I sincerely thank you for understanding the essence of my discovery that hyperventilation is a cause of those diseases.

I wish you success in popularising this discovery — even after 44 years I could not reach all the people in the world with it, mainly because of medical conservatism.

With respect,
Professor Buteyko

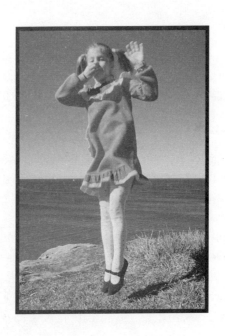

Some Common Questions About the Method, and the Answers

⭐ I want to know whether I am one of the hidden hyperventilators that the Professor talks about. How can I find out?

Sit down and breathe through the nose for two minutes. Breathe out completely, squeeze your nose to block it and hold your breath while timing yourself with a watch that has a second hand.

At the first sign of breath hunger, start breathing again, and write down the time achieved. If you achieve 15 seconds, then you are a hidden hyperventilator and are breathing for four people.

If you achieve 30 seconds you are breathing for two people.

If you achieve 50–60 seconds before experiencing the first difficulty, then you are not a hidden hyperventilator, and are breathing for one person.

⭐ You mention carbon dioxide a lot in this book. What about oxygen? How much do we need in our lungs, and what other gases are present too? Does the method affect the amount of these that we breathe in and out, and if so what are the effects?

The composition of air is 20.93% oxygen, 0.03% carbon dioxide and 79.04% nitrogen. Having read the chapter on the physiology of breathing, you will know that our lungs create an atmospheric environment different from that of the outside air. Inside our lungs, the normal atmosphere comprises 14% oxygen, 6% carbon dioxide, 75% nitrogen and 5% water vapour. The oxygen we breathe in is more than adequate for our needs, and most of it is breathed out again (this means that we can revive another person, if necessary, by breathing our own air into his or her lungs). But the carbon dioxide is precious, because it needs to be at the right level so that the oxygen can be released from the blood and made available to the body tissues.

★ **If 90% of the population over-breathes, and over-breathing causes asthma, why do we not all have asthma?**

Over-breathing, according to the Buteyko theory, is the hidden cause of a number of illnesses. Because we all have different bodies, we have different vulnerability towards diseases. People who develop asthma as a result of over-breathing have what is termed a 'tendency' towards respiratory disorders, that is, they are more likely to succumb to them when they are placed at risk by a deterioration in their general health.

★ **Are there any health conditions that would make it dangerous or impossible for someone to do the Buteyko method?**

No, provided they are taught by a practitioner. However, patients with severe angina or hypertension must only do control pauses at first, and must not attempt the maximum pause until they have achieved some improvement under the guidance of their Buteyko practitioner and doctor.

⭐ I am a diver, and I and my fellow divers hyperventilate for some time before free diving, to store oxygen. Is it harmful to do this? It helps me stay down longer.

If you are a fit person and you hyperventilate for a brief period before a dive, this will not effect your general fitness, and it will help you to take more oxygen on board. Remember that if you have learned the Buteyko method this will increase your fitness even more, and build up more reserve. After all, diving means that you are practising the Buteyko maximum pause, underwater. Beware, however, that if someone has a tendency to asthma, angina, emphysema or anxiety, hyperventilating in the way you describe could bring on an attack.

⭐ If you learn the Buteyko exercises for the treatment of asthma, does that mean you have to continue them for the rest of your life?

In mild asthma, after two to three months the breathing becomes reconditioned back to normal — that is, the asthma sufferer learns to breathe for one person. Usually the person does not have to continue the exercises, except when they have a virus or are under some other severe stress. Remember, Buteyko practitioners say that one maximum pause equals two puffs of a bronchodilator at the onset of an attack. If the maximum pause does not work, then the puffer can be used. People with moderate to severe asthma need to carry on with the exercises indefinitely if they want to control their asthma naturally.

☆ My little girl would be frightened of holding her breath in the way you describe — it is not easy to teach her things, or even to get her to take her asthma medication properly. So how can the Buteyko method help her?

If your girl is over four-and-a-half years old, she is able to do the method. Children find the exercises fun and get quite competitive with one another. If your girl is under four, you can start with reminding her to breathe through the nose and encouraging her to only sleep on her left side. You can also book her into a swimming class, as a preliminary to her learning the Buteyko method.

☆ I am a mild asthmatic, but I play the flute, and find that asthma does not interfere with my flute playing. Why is this?

In mild asthma the slight hyperventilation due to the flute playing will cause few if any problems. However, you would have better control and hold your notes longer if you underwent tuition under a Buteyko practitioner. Also, in sustaining long notes you are actually following part of the Buteyko technique.

⭐ Is there a way I can measure the amount of air I breathe by using my peak flow meter?

No, these meters measure peak expiratory flow, not the volume of air breathed per minute.

⭐ Do you have any advice on encouraging a child to sleep in the beneficial way you describe?

Help your child to settle comfortably on the left side when he or she gets into bed. To encourage breathing through the nose, first be assured that your child's nasal passages are normally free, then you can begin by partially taping up the mouth with micropore tape. This is not frightening for a child, because it can be pulled off very easily, and it does not cause discomfort or allergy. When the child is used to the partial taping, the mouth can be fully taped until breathing through the nose becomes normal during sleep.

⭐ I am pregnant, and in my antenatal relaxation classes I am told to breathe deeply. Is this harmful?

All forms of deep breathing can cause anxiety, asthma or angina, particularly in people prone to those conditions. In severe deep breathing, especially if rapid, the smooth muscles around the blood vessels to the placenta can become narrowed (go into spasm), and this is potentially dangerous to the baby.

✪ None of my children has asthma, but I am always worried that one of them will get it, as pollution is high where I live. Should I teach them your breathing exercises as a preventative?

Pollution can cause irritation to the airways because of toxicity and allergy. These alone can lead to asthma, but a lowered resistance to infection due to pollution is another cause. An increasing number of people are developing asthma for the first time after a severe virus or series of viruses. Pollution is one of the main triggers that cause over-breathing, which can be corrected by the Buteyko method. As always, one should be taught by a trained practitioner.

✪ My baby is only one year old, but he has been diagnosed with asthma. Is there anything I can do to help him breathe properly, or must I wait until he is old enough to learn the method?

It is impossible to teach breathing techniques to a child at one year of age. Apart from using orthodox drug therapy you can improve his nutrition with vitamins and herbs (see the chapter on diet in this book). Overfeeding a baby is not good for him, but demand feeding will do no harm. When you put your child to bed, help him to get comfortable on his left side, as this is the most beneficial position for breathing. Do not tape up the mouths of a babies or small children if they breathe through their mouths when asleep — they can be taught to breathe through the nose when they are older.

☆ How can I find out more about the Buteyko technique and the Buteyko practitioners?

Here are some telephone numbers for Buteyko.

Sydney, Australia:

(Free call within Australia only)

Hastings, New Zealand:

London, England:

Dublin, Ireland:

Bethlehem, USA:

Australian website for Buteyko:

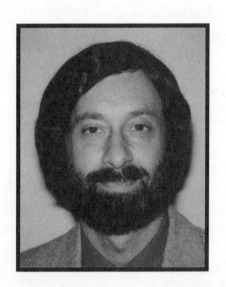

Acknowledgments

From the Author

My thanks go to Professor K.P. Buteyko who conceived and utilised a brilliant and basic theory — that hyperventilation is the cause of some 150 medical conditions. I thank Sasha Stalmatsky who taught and guided all of us in 'the Method', Christopher Drake who put the Buteyko method on the map, Jac Vidgen, a great public speaker and teacher of the method and Rosalba Belford for her energy and advice in the nutrition chapter. Special thanks also to Tess Graham for her fortitude and determination in carrying out the clinical trials, keeping them true to the end. I would also like to thank ACNEM, the Australian College of Nutritional and Environmental Medicine.

My appreciation also to Annette Ameisen, who single-handedly typed and correlated my notes and gave me continuous support, Nancy Hollander, who expertly and enthusiastically photographed the Buteyko exercises, Lola and Vera Motina for their help during the photographic sessions and my children Belinda and Abigayle for their enthusiastic modelling.

I would like to thank Maggie Hamilton of Bantam Books who gave sound advice and helped with editing.

For her encouragement, continued belief in the book, creative editing and advice, I thank Cheryl Hingley.

Finally, for her support, patience and encouragement, I thank Suzi Grgurevic.

From the Publisher

The Publisher would like to thank the following for giving permission to reproduce material from publications or advertisements: Astra Australia; *Australian Doctor* and Tony James; *Medical Observer*; News Limited (Katrina Beikoff and Natalie Williams); Rebecca Thurlow, *The Sun Herald* (April 13, 1997); TIME Magazine.

Grateful thanks are due to Christopher Drake in Dublin and Russell and Jenny Stark in New Zealand for their assistance with information on the Buteyko method in the UK and New Zealand. Thanks also to Aaron Lumsdaine for information on Buteyko in the USA.

Index

*Italic page numbers refer
to illustrations*

acupuncture 141
advertising *see* marketing
air sacs 89, 90–1
Aitken, Jonathan 171–2
'Alan' 59–60
alcohol 131, 132
   and recreational drugs 24,
      103
Aldecin MDI 119
Alexander technique 142
alkalosis 89
allergies 132–5
alternative treatments 127–43
Alupent MDI 109
alveoli 89, 90–1
Ameisen, Paul J. *12, 154*
Aminophylline 123
anaphylaxis 123
angina sufferers 184–5
'Anne' 65–8
antibiotics 122–3
anticholinergic bronchodilators
      108, 109
   side effects 111–12
antihistamines 124
anti-inflammatories 108, 117,
      119

aromatherapy 143
Asmol MDI 109
asthma
   alleviation of symptoms 31
   death rate 8, 116–17
   inciidence in Australia 7, 8
   incidence in NZ 7, 168
   incidence in UK 8, 171
   incidence in USA 7, 115
   naturopathy and 127–43
Asthma and Respiratory
      Foundation, New Zealand
      168, 169
Asthma Foundation of Victoria
   early warnings against
      Buteyko method 32–3, 159
Asthma Foundations,
      Australian 8, 34, 158, 161
Asthma Societies, New
      Zealand 169
athletes 21
Atrovent MDI 109
auscultation 146
Australia 155–67
Australian Association of
      Asthma Foundations 161
Australian Buteyko
      Association formed 158
Australian College of Nutritional
      and Environmental
      Medicine 166

Australian Doctor 113, 118, 162–3, 165
Australian Medical Acupuncture Society 166
Austyn caps 123

babies 188
  see also children
'Barbara' 77–8
B complex vitamins 136, 137
Becloforte MDI 119
Beclomethasone 119
Becotide MDI 119
Becotide Rotacaps 119
Belford, Rosalba 158
'Bernard' 84–5
Berotec MDI 109
Beta-agonist bronchodilators 108, 109
  dangers 112–17
  side effects 111
bioflavonoids 135–6
blood, oxygenation of 92–3, 94–5
BOHR effect 94–5
Booth, Ginny 176–7
Bowler, Simon 11, 161, 164
breathing levels 18, 24, 97, 103
breathing physiology 87–103
Brezezinski, Matthew and Brandon 179
Bricanyl elixir 109
Bricanyl MDI 109
Bricanyl tabs 109
Bricanyl Turbuhaler 109

Brighthope, Ian 166
bronchodilators 23, 102–3, 108, 109–17
  long-acting 117
  reduced use in Buteyko method 124–5, 167
  replacing with maximum pause 43
  side effects 111–12
Brondecon expectorant and elixir 123
Brondecon PD tabs 123
Bryan's cytotoxic test 135
Budesonide 119
Buteyko, Konstantin Pavlovich 8–9, *144*, 145–6, 180–1
  clinical studies 149–52
Buteyko Institute for Breathing and Health Inc 175
Buteyko method 15–27
  as alternative to drugs 124–5
  in Australia 155–67
  favourable results 45–85, 176–9
  length of treatment 34, 37, 185–6
  in New Zealand 168–71
  practising 29–43
  reduced drug intake 10, 11, 124–5, 167
  in Russia 145–53
  technique 34–5
  typical session 41
  in United Kingdom 171–3
  in United States 173–9

Buteyko USA Ltd 179

candidiasis 120, 121
carbon dioxide 16–17, 87–89,
    92–3, 96, 183–4
Cardophyllin suppositories
    123
'Catherine' 47–8, 57
Chi gong 142, 166
children
    improved behaviour 125
    learning the Buteyko
        method 186, 187
chiropractic 141
chocolate 132
Choledyl tabs 123
cholesterol production 20
Choline theophyllinate 123
'Christana' 78–81
clinical trials
    Queensland 10–11, 160–7
    Russia 149–52
    Victoria 160
coffee and tea 131, 132
control pause 36, 40, 42–3, 51
cooked food 102, 128, 131
Corticosteroids 108, 119
Cortisone acetate 119
Crane, Julian 168–9

Daily Mail 172
Daily Telegraph Mirror 120–1
deep breathing
    belief in 21, 93, 101
    research 146–8

diet and nutrition 22, 101–2,
    128–32
Diproprionate 119
diseases resulting from over-
    breathing 19, 98–9
diving, hyperventilating before
    185
'Dominic' 64–5
Drake, Christopher 156, 157,
    171, 172–3, 174
Dr Coca test 133–4
drugs see medication; alcohol
    and recreational drugs
dysphonia 121

electrodermal testing 134–5
Elixophyllin elixir 123
'Emma' 76–7
emphysema 32
exercise 22, 102, 138–40

Fenoterol 109, 114
fish, dietary 129, 130
flute playing 186

'Giovanna' 76
glucocorticoids 117
Graham, Tess 11, 161
Green, Amanda 161

haemoglobin 92, 93, 94
hay fever 31–2
Heffner, Richard 176
herbal treatment 140
hidden hyperventilation 17,

96, 183
Holm, Paige 179
homoeopathic agents 140
hot and stuffy environments
    23, 102
hypertension sufferers 184–5
hyperventilation *see* over-
    breathing
hypoglycaemia 129
hypothalamic pituitary adrenal
    axis depression 120–1
hypoxia 93

illness *see* diseases;
    side effects; over-
    breathing, results of
inflammation (swelling) of
    mucus lining and bronchial
    tubes 10, 20, 100, 116
Intal 122
Intal Forte MDI 119
Intal MDI 119
Intal Spincaps 119
Ipratropium bromide 109

'Jane' 61–2
'Joan'and her husband
    68–73
'Joshua' 83–4

'Kelly' 47
Kerr, Caleb 178
leukotrienne antagonist 120

Listen machine 134–5

Lister, Joseph 148–9
'Lola' 62–3
low-stress diet 129, 131
Lumsdaine, Aaron 173–5, 179
lung structure 88, 90–1

magnesium 136
magnesium sulphate 137
manganese deficiency 128–9
marketing of bronchodilators
    112–13, 115
massage and aromatherapy
    143
MAST cell inhibitors 136
maximum pause 36–7, 40, 42,
    43
    prolonging 39–40, *52–5*
meat, dietary 102, 128
media coverage of Buteyko
    method 157, 172
Medical Observer 138–9
medication (drugs) 107–25
    cases of reduction 63, 65–6,
        77–8, 79, 83, 84–5
    for mild asthma 46
    monitoring 29–30, 33
    reducing 33–4
Medocromil 119, 122
Meshalkin, Professor 146, 149,
    150–1
micropore tape 35, *50*, 187
mild asthma 37–8, 46
    favourable Buteyko results
        47–8, 57–9
minerals and vitamins 135–7

Mitchell, Charles 11, 161, 164–5
moderate asthma 38, 59
favourable Buteyko results 59–74
Mora test 134–5
mucolytics 124
mucus and phlegm production 10, 20, 100, 116
muscles 93

naturopathy 127–43
negative ion therapy 143
New Zealand 168–71
nitrogen 183–4
Nuelin sprinkle 123
Nuelin SR 123
Nuelin syrup 123
Nuelin tabs 123
nutrition and diet 22, 101–2, 128–32

O'Byrne, Paul *118*
Odhner, Catherine 177
Odhner, Patricia 176
Orciprenaline 109
osteopathy 141
osteoporosis 125
over-breathing (hyper-ventilation) 9–10, 16, 96, 104, 184
    defense mechanisms 10, 99–101, 115–16
    method of detecting 183
    results of 17–21, 26–7, 98–9
    triggers 21–4, 101–3
over-eating 22, 101–2, 128
oxygen 183–4
oxygen starvation 17, 92–3, 95

Parnell, Gregory 157
peak flow meters 40, 187
pollution 24, 188
Prednisolone 119
Prednisone 119
pregnancy 187
preventatives 117–24
primum non nocere principle 30
puffers *see* bronchodilators
Pulmicort MDI 119
Pulmicort Turbuhaler 119

quercetin 136

RAST test 133
Reader, Mabel 178
respiratory alkalosis 89
respiratory disorder tendency 184
Respolin MDI 109
Rupp, Ira 178

Salbutamol 109, 114
Salmeterol 109
Salmeterol Xinafoate 117
Saskatchewan Asthma Epidemiology Project 114
Schecter, Gloria 176

selenium 136
Semmelweiss, Ignaz Philipp
148–9
Serevent 117
Serevent disks 109
Serevent MDI 109
severe asthma 38, 75
favourable Buteyko results
75–85
sexual activity, excessive 23–4,
103
shallow breathing 21, 42, 43,
49, 95–6, 105
Shiatsu 142
side effects
antibiotics 122–3
bronchodilators 111–12
steroids 118–21
Xanthines 122
sinusitis 31
Sio-Bid caps 123
skin prick test 133
sleep
on left side 35, 50, 187, 188
prolonged and excessive
22–3, 102
sleep apnoea 32
smoking and tobacco 24, 103,
131, 132
snoring 32
Sodium cromoglycate 108,
119, 122
spasm of the airways and air
sacs 10, 20, 100, 116
spicy foods 129

Stalmatsky, Alexander 'Sasha'
155, 155–6, 161, 171,
174
Stark, Russell and Jennifer 168,
170
steroids 117–21
side effects 118–21
stress 22, 101
stress reduction and rest
137–8
sugar 132
Sunday Telegraph 82
Sun Herald 74–5
swimming 21, 126, 138–40
symptoms of over-breathing
19, 20, 26–7, 98–9

Tai chi 142, 166
taping the mouth 35, 50
not advised for babies 188
partial 187
Tareiev, Evengly Mikhailovitch
146
tea and coffee 131, 132
Terbutaline 109
Theo-Dur tabs 123
Theophylline 123
Thera test 134–5
Thompson, Sarah 168
Thoracic Society of Australia
and New Zealand
Annual Scientific Meeting,
Hobart (1995) 11, 163
Tilade 119, 122
Time magazine 110

tobacco and smoking 24, 103, 131, 132
Tracey, Kevin 157
treatment, choosing 30–5
Triplett, Danielle 177–8

United Kingdom 171–3
United States of America 173–9
USSR Academy of Science, Siberian Branch
  Institute of Cytology and Genetics 151, 152

Vega test 134–5
Ventolin MDI 109
Ventolin Rotocaps 109
Ventolin syrup 109
Ventolin tabs 109

'Vera' 57–8
VERIGO-BOHR effect 94–5
Vidgen, Jac 174
vitamin A 136
vitamin B complex 136, 137
vitamin C 135, 137
vitamin D 136
vitamin E 136
vitamin injection 137
vitamins and minerals 135–7

water, drinking 132
Wiley-Nieves, Guines 177

Xanthines 108, 122, 123

yoga 142–3

zinc 136

FORM 1

LAKE CARRIERS' ASSOCIATION
IDENTIFICATION CARD

NOV 2 2 1934

For Steamer *Gordoil*

Lying at *Shell Oil Dock River Rouge*

Recommended as *Watchman*

LAKE CARRIERS'
ASSOCIATION

NOV 2 2 1934

ASSEMBLY ROOM,
DETROIT

J W Westcott J.
Commissioner

Left office at *11 40 Pm*

Murdanie MacLeod
Signature of Applicant

Discharge Book No. *103179*, which is in his possession and must be presented with this card.

Form 978.

SERIAL NUMBER
190006

UNITED STATES
DEPARTMENT OF COMMERCE
STEAMBOAT INSPECTION SERVICE

FILE No. 8 *6557*

CERTIFICATE OF SERVICE TO ABLE SEAMAN.

This is to certify that *Murdanie MacLeod* *27* years of age, born in *Scotland*, having given satisfactory evidence to the undersigned United States Local Inspectors, Steamboat Inspection Service, for the district of *Buffalo, N.Y.*, that he has had the experience required by law, to all of which proof is made by affidavit, and having passed the examination as to eyesight, hearing, and physical condition prescribed by the Department of Commerce, is hereby rated as an Able Seaman for service on the *High seas and any inland waters*

Issued by the undersigned Board of Local Inspectors on this *7th* day of *July* 193*1*.

Signature of able seaman:

Murdanie MacLeod

James M. Foy
William P. Nolen
U. S. Local Inspectors.

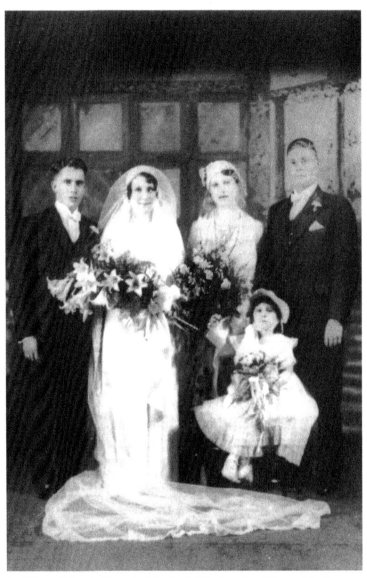
An Uig wedding in Detroit, Murdanie MacLeod and Peggy MacLennan

No. 112341

Marriage License

Wayne County, Michigan

193_2_

To any person legally authorised to solemnize marriage,

Greeting:

Marriage May Be Solemnized Between

Mr. __Murdanie MacLeod__ and M __Peggy MacLennan__,

affidavit having been filed in this office, as provided by Public Act No. 128, Laws of 1887, as amended, by which it appears that said

__Murdanie MacLeod__ is __29__ years of age,

color is __white__, residence is __Detroit, Michigan__, and birthplace was __Scotland__, occupation is __auto worker__, father's name __Donald__, and mother's maiden name was __Isabella__

has been previously married __no__ time s ; and that said __Peggy MacLennan__

is __31__ years of age, color is __white__ residence is __Detroit, Michigan__ and birthplace was __Scotland__ occupation is __waitress__, father's name __Murdo__, and mother's maiden name was __Annie MacAulay__

and who has been previously married __no__ time s , and whose maiden name was

____, and whose ____ consent, in case she
Parent's or Guardian's

has not attained the age of eighteen years, has been filed in my office.

In Witness Whereof, I have hereunto attached my hand and the seal of Wayne County, Michigan, this __12th__

[L. S.] day of __September__ A. D. 193 2.

Thos F Farrell
County Clerk

by _Cass J. Hill_
D Dfuty Clerk   HP

Certificate of Marriage

Between Mr. _Murdanie MacLeod_ and M _Peggy MacLennan_

I hereby certify that, in accordance with the above license, the persons herein mentioned were joined in marriage by me, at _Detroit_, County of _Wayne_, Michigan,

on the _22nd_ day of _September_ A. D. 193_2_, in the presence

of _Isabella Macdonald_, of _Detroit_,

and _Detroit Donald Morrison_, of _Detroit_,

as witnesses.

Roy L. Aldrich
Name of Magistrate or clergyman

Minister
Official Title

THIS DUPLICATE must be delivered by the person solemnizing marriage to one of the parties joined in marriage.

BIBLIOGRAPHY

Highland history

The Making of the Crofting Community: James Hunter (John Donald)

The Islands of Scotland: Hugh MacDiarmid (Batsford)

Old Statistical Account

New Statistical Account

Canna: The Story of a Hebridean Island: J. L. Campbell (Oxford University Press)

History of the Highland Clearances (Vols I and I I): Eric Richards

History of the Mathesons: A. MacKenzie and A. MacBain (MacKay)

Lewis: A History of the Island: Donald MacDonald (Gordon Wright)

The Hebrides: W. H. Murray (Heinemann)

Harris and Lewis: Francis Thompson (David and Charles: Islands Series)

The People's Clearance: J. M. Bumstead (Edinburgh University Press)

A History of Scotland: J. D. Mackie (Pelican)

The Highland Clearances: A. Mackenzie (A. MacLaren)

The Highland Clearances: John Prebble (Secker and Warburg)

History of the Outer Hebrides: W. C. Mackenzie (A. Gardner)

Public Administration in the Highlands and Islands: J. P. Day (University of London Press)

The Isle of Lewis and Harris: Arthur Geddes

The Highlands and Islands of Scotland: W. C. Mackenzie (Moray Press)

Crofting Years: Frank Thompson (Luath Press)

Skye and the Outer Hebrides: W. Douglas Simpson (Robert Hale)

Tong: The Story of a Lewis Village: Tong History Society
Surprise Island: James Shaw Grant (James Thin)

Scottish/American history

The Scots Overseas: Gordon Donaldson (Robert Hale)
Colonists from Scotland: Emigration to North America (1707–83) (Cornell University Press)
Directory of Scottish Settlers in America (1625–1825): David Dobson (Genealogical Publishing)
The Emigrant Scots: Michael Brander (Constable)
Highland Settler: The Scottish Gael in Nova Scotia: Charles Dunn (University of Toronto)
The Highland Scots in North Carolina: Meyer (Chapel Hill)
Scotus Americanus: William R. Brock (Edinburgh University Press)
Colonists from Scotland: Graham (Kennikat Press)

Emigration (General)

Immigrant Groups in Canada: ed. Elliot (Prentice Hall)
British Immigrants in Industrial America: Berthoff (Harvard University Press)
Immigrants: Harvey and Troper (Von Nostrand Reinhold)
Emigration from the British Isles: Carrothers (P. S. King and Son)
The Search for Prosperity: Richard Garret (Wayland)

Canada and USA

The Roar of the Twenties: James H. Gray
Detroit: ed. Holli (Franklin Watts)
Social Welfare in Ontario (1791–1893): Richard Splane (University of Toronto Press)
Historical Statistics of Canada: Urquhart and Buckley (Cambridge MacMillan)

American Ethnic Groups: Cordasco and Alloway (Scarecrow)
Farmer Premier: The Memoirs of E. C. Drury: (McLelland and Stewart)

Leverhulme

Viscount Leverhulme by his Son (George Allen and Unwin)
Lord Leverhulme: W. P. Jolly
Lord of the Isles: Nigel Nicholson

Opium War and Far East

Foreign Mud: Maurice Collis (Faber and Faber)
The Opium War: Brian Inglis (Coronet)
British Trade With China (Pamphlet): James Matheson (Smith Elder and Co.)
The East India Company: Brian Gardner (Hart Davis)

Shipping

Canadian Pacific Afloat (CPR in Association with the World Ship Society)
Merchant Fleets in Profile: Duncan Haws (Patrick Stephens)
Great Passenger Ships of the World: Arnold Kludas (Patrick Stephens)

Journals

West Highland Mercenaries in Ireland: Andrew McKerral (Scottish Historical Review Vol. XXX, 1951)
James Matheson of the Lews: A. MacKenzie (Celtic Magazine, 1882 and Private Pamphlet)

Songs

Eilean nan Fhraoich: Songs of Lewis (Acair)

Parliamentary Papers

Overseas Settlement: House of Commons Reports: 1919, 1920, 1921, 1922, 1923, 1924, 1925. Report of Committee: 1923. Empire Settlement Act: 1922.
Landholders Acts: 1886–1919
Scottish Land Court Reports: Vol. VIII (1919), Vol. XI (1923)
Brand Report: 1902

Others

Highland Journey: Colin MacDonald
I Crossed the Minch: Louis MacNeice (Longman)
New York Telephone Directories

Newspapers consulted

West Highland Free Press
Stornoway Gazette
People's Journal
Glasgow Herald
The Scotsman
Edinburgh Courant
London Evening News
Toronto Star
Toronto Globe
Toronto Telegram
St John Daily Telegraph
The Bulletin
Eilean nan Fhraoich magazine